Positive Affirmations

Learn the Power of Positive Affirmations for Self Healing, Good Health, Weight Loss, Wealth, Success, Money, Prosperity, a Better Life & Teach it to Your Kids. For Men & Women

Dr. Louise Lily Wain

All effort has been executed to present accurate, up to date, and reliable, complete information. No warranties of any kind are declared or implied.

Readers acknowledge that the author is not engaging in the rendering of legal, financial, medical or professional advice.

The content within this book has been derived from various sources.

Please consult a licensed professional before attempting any techniques outlined in this book.

By reading this document, the reader agrees that under no circumstances is the author responsible for any losses, direct or indirect, which are incurred as a result of the use of the information contained within this document, including, but not limited to, — errors, omissions, or inaccuracies.

Table of Contents

Introduction

Do you desire to enjoy the enormous benefits of this book "POSITIVE AFFIRMATIONS"?

Then keep reading as I unravel all you need to know about positive affirmations.

As humans, mental stability is very vital.

Having a good understanding of positive thinking is a key component that allows individuals, groups of persons or entire societies to flourish in this present day.

Positive thinking plays a vital role in the way humans grow, succeed and maintain stable well-being.

Situations characterized by positive emotions can as well constitute to a higher positive affirmation.

The following under listed are reasons why your positive affirmations do not work for you and what you can do to ensure that they work for you to assist you to achieve your goals and maximize your potential within your most vital roles. :

- ➤ You are not being realistic with your affirmations
- ➤ You do have the Feeling that you are Lying to Yourself
- ➤ You are Just Going Through the Motions
- ➤ You are not saying it appropriately

➢ Your Positive Affirmations are too many
➢ You are exceeding your limits

Ideal ways to practice positive affirmations

The following are ways to say your affirmations and make them work for you.

➢ Saying the affirmations utilizing a confident tone, such as you sincerely believe what you are saying.
➢ Standing in a relaxed, upright position in which your body is in a perfect posture
➢ Saying the affirmations with a positive mindset and having the belief that they must work
➢ Saying it out loud
➢ Saying the affirmations one at a time, slowly and deliberately
➢ Saying them by watching yourself in the mirror; as seeing yourself so relaxed, positive and hopeful creates a positive loop in which you are confident in what you are saying more, and then you are more comfortable with it.

In this book; "POSITIVE AFFIRMATIONS", there are some benefits to obtain after reading such as:

➢ Dealing with negative thoughts
➢ How to use positive affirmations effectively

- ➢ The best way to recite positive affirmations
- ➢ How often to recite affirmations
- ➢ How to create your own positive affirmations
- ➢ How to teach affirmation to your kids
- ➢ A list of affirmations for kid's e.t.c.

Chapter 1

What are Positive Affirmations

The manner we utilize in talking to ourselves as well as others shapes how we feel about ourselves.

You will not feel good if you are negative to yourself and therefore the people in your life.

Positive affirmations set you free from fear, guilt, anxiety, negativity, and pain.

These mantras are simply easy messages that when repeated over-and-over, begin to percolate into your mind; slowly changing both your thinking and your reality.

Sometimes these sayings begin as wishful thinking, but they usually end up becoming the reality of your life.

Affirmations are positive statements that can assist you to challenge and defeat self-sabotaging and negative thoughts.

When you repeat them regularly and believe them, you will begin to invite some positive changes.

You might view affirmations to be unrealistic "wishful thinking."

But try viewing positive affirmations this way: myriads of folks do repetitive exercises to enhance their physical health, and affirmations are like exercises for our mind and appearance.

These positive mental repetitions can reprogram our thinking patterns so that, over time, we begin to think and act distinctively.

Self-affirmation can as well assist to mitigate the consequences of stress.

The Way to Utilize Positive Affirmations

The following are ways to utilize positive affirmations:

Pay attention to the present.

Write down your positive affirmation in the present tense rather than future-focused.

For instance, "I am healthy" rather than "I am going to be healthy".

Writing your statements in this way assists your subconscious mind to believe it is already occurring.

This will naturally assist ease the transition from affirming to doing.

It also assists your brain to create positive feelings related to your required change and this reward will definitely encourage your continued practice.

Affirmations using the first person.

Write down your affirmation with "I" rather than "you".

For instance, "I am excited" instead of "You are excited".

This assists instill a stronger sense of identity in the brain.

You can as well include your name if that is helpful.

Find out what you want to change.

Begin by making an inventory of the areas of your life where you would like to witness changes happen.

You can as well make an inventory of the areas that are going well and that you would like to see continue.

Is it a desired emotion you would like to feel more regularly?

Changes in your environment?

An attitude you want to let go of?

Whatever the case may be, add it to your list.

Now circle your top five desired areas.

From this smaller list choose just one area as your beginning focus.

You can at any time return to the present list once you want to practice other positive affirmations.

Always be smart.

As with any goal, the most successful aspirations ought to be Specific, Achievable or Actionable, Measurable, Realistic, and Timely.

Even if your unique positive affirmation does not meet all of those criteria it is vital to keep it as focused as possible.

This will assist create a very specific image in your mind's eye which is attainable in the real world.

Produce a well-detailed image.

Include the previous steps into an in-depth visualization of your positive affirmation to keep in your mind's eye while you state your mantra.

Be specific on where you are and the person you are with but most significantly focus the way you feel.

Remember, your feelings are the best motivating factor toward your required goal.

Do some practice regularly.

As with any desired change, whether it is breaking an unwanted habit or learning a new skill such as playing an instrument, "practice they say makes perfect".

The more often you practice your positive affirmation the stronger your brain rewires itself to simply accept these mantras as true.

Be careful of triggers.

There could be some positive affirmations you are not prepared to hear.

For some persons, utilizing kind words towards themselves can actually be too painful.

This is often the case if abusive words were heard during childhood.

For instance, the positive affirmation "I am worthy" can actually make some persons feel worse because it is going to be unlocking painful memories where they were made to feel the other.

Pay an Attention to the Positive.

To increase the likelihood of success it is vital to state your affirmation as a positive sentence instead of employing a negative sentence structure.

The brain focuses on keywords instead of a full sentence; so, if you make the statement "I am not weak" your brain will ultimately focus on that word "weak.

It is therefore ideal to rephrase this as the positive statement "I am strong".

Link the feeling to the behavior.

Desired behaviors that are linked to positive feelings are more likely to turn into real actions.

This is due to the fact that pleasure acts as a reward that you will want to repeat again and again.

For instance, "I get up for myself and I feel empowered" instead of "I get up for myself".

The feeling word "empowered" gives strength to the affirmation.

These abusive alterations that are negative can feel more truthful than any positive affirmation.

If this is often the case it is going to take longer to believe your positive affirmations but that is ok.

Pace yourself, stop as required if it becomes too painful, use a special mantra, and return to the first positive affirmation once you are ready.

There is no rush, so take your time and be kind to yourself as much as possible.

Make use of an app.

We are lucky that technology is available to assist us to obtain our personal development goals!

There are many smartphone apps to enhance your practice. (See page 40 for list of positive affirmation apps)

Get the most out of technology.

An alternative means to harness technology for your practice is to utilize the tools already installed on your Smartphone.

> ➤ When you have developed a personalized affirmation, record it by utilizing the voice memo feature. Listen to your affirmation several times in the entire day.

- ➢ Set a reminder which will appear frequently on your Phone screen.
- ➢ Set a notification to sound each hour, and have your affirmation repeated when you hear the ring.

Find the best way to practice for you.

There is no single way to practice positive affirmations.

You may want to create your personal mantras, or you may want to utilize other person's words.

The key is to ensure you schedule a constant practice, visualize your positive affirmation as vividly as possible, and check out to feel the mantra take hold in your body.

How To Write an Affirmation Statement

Affirmation statements often target a selected area, behavior or belief that you are battling with.

The following points can assist you to write the affirmation statement that best fits your needs.

Ensure that your affirmation is credible and can be achieved.

It should be based on a realistic assessment of the facts.

For example, imagine that you are not happy with the level of money that you currently earn.

You could utilize affirmations to raise your confidence to request a raise.

However, it probably would not be wise to affirm to yourself that you are going to double your salary: for most persons, and most organizations, doubling what you are earning in one go is not very feasible.

Keep it real; After all, affirmations are not magic spells.

If you cannot believe in them, it is unlikely they will impact your life.

Transform negatives to positives.

If you are battling with negative self-talk, note down the persistent thoughts or beliefs that are disturbing you.

Then choose an affirmation that is the opposite of that thought and belief.

For instance, if you habitually think, "I'm not talented enough to make progress in my career," turn this around and write a positive affirmation like, "I am a skilled and experienced professional."

Note the areas of your life that you would like to change.

For example, do you wish that you had more patience?

Or deeper relationships with your friends and colleagues?

Or would you prefer a more productive workday?

Write down several areas or behaviors that you would like to work on.

Ensure that they are compatible with your core values and the things that matter the most to you so that you will feel genuinely motivated to achieve them.

Affirm it with feeling.

Affirmations are often simpler once they carry emotional weight.

You need to require this change to occur, so every affirmation that you simply prefer to repeat should be a phrase that is meaningful to you.

For instance, if you are worried about a new project that you have been tasked with, you could tell yourself, "I am really happy to take on new challenges."

Your affirmation must be in the present tense.

Write and speak your affirmation as if it is already occurring.

This assists you to believe that the statement is true right now.

For example, "I am well-prepared and well-rehearsed, and I can offer a great presentation" would be a great affirmation to make use of if you feel nervous speaking in front of a group.

Why Use Positive Affirmations

Successful individuals, from top salespeople and entrepreneurs to bestselling authors and Olympic athletes, have found out that using willpower to power their success is certainly not enough.

You need to abandon any negative thoughts and pictures and bombard your subconscious mind with recent thoughts and pictures that are positive and stated in the present tense.

The way to do this

The technique you utilize to do this is referred to as daily affirmations, which is simply a statement that describes a goal in its already completed state.

Two instances of affirmations would be:

> ➤ I am happily walking across the stage as I receive my MBA degree.
> ➤ I am so excited and thankful that I am now crossing the finishing line of the Marathon.

Repeating daily affirmations assists to reprogram the unconscious mind for success.

It assists to get rid of negative and limiting beliefs and transforms your comfort zone from a limited one keeping you trapped in mediocrity to a more expanded one where anything is feasible.

It assists to replace your "I cant's" with "I cans," and your fears and doubts with more confidence and certainty.

The Way Daily Affirmations Keep You Focused

Daily affirmations are simply reminders to your unconscious mind to place your eyes on your goals and to come up with solutions to combat obstacles that might get in the way.

Daily affirmations as well can create higher vibrations of happiness, joy, appreciation, and gratitude that then, through the law of attraction, magnetize individuals, resources, and opportunities to come to you to assist you to achieve your goals.

Create Recent Daily Positive Affirmations for Yourself

Write down three affirmations for yourself that affirm you having already achieved three of your goals and dreams.

Then, write down the time of the day that you will commit to practicing your affirmations.

Is it when you wake up from bed in the morning?

Before you go to bed?

Or during mid-day when you need a pick-me-up?

Chapter 2

Importance of Self Talk

Self-talk is what you do naturally throughout the time you are not asleep.

A lot of persons are getting more aware that positive self-talk may be a powerful tool for increasing your self-confidence and preventing negative emotions.

Individuals that can get more acquainted with positive self-talk are thought to be a lot more confident, productive, and motivated.

Although positive self-talk comes naturally to some, most persons got to find out how to cultivate positive thoughts and dispel the negative ones.

With practice, it can become more natural to think good thoughts instead of bad ones.

Self Talk is an enormous part of what makes us who we are.

It has an impact on how we feel about ourselves, how we feel about what we will achieve in life, how we are seen by the planet and the way we interact with other persons. It also impacts our self-esteem, self-confidence, and self-image.

Most folks express some sort of negative self-talk also as external talk towards ourselves.

We get the knowledge from our caregivers, and then perpetuate it for a lot of years creating who we are.

Observing how we talk to ourselves is the beginning of changing it for the better.

You are the one that controls every aspect of your life.

Talking to yourself – finding the emotions, emotions, and thoughts that guide you is the blueprint of your impact on the planet.

This will govern the standard of the life you have got for yourself.

The same actions and circumstances may occur to 2 persons but it is how you talk to yourself that will decide how your life continues from then.

Some will take a more negative route where other persons would utilize it and make a positive action to better their lives.

You need to make the selection of which way it will go, and make it the simplest outcome you most likely can.

Ensure you recognize the language of yourself, and tell yourself a positive story and go on an adventure only for you.

How to utilize self-talk on a daily basis

Positive self-talk requires some practice if it is not your natural instinct.

If you are generally more pessimistic, you can practice shifting your inner dialogue to be more encouraging and uplifting.

However, forming a replacement habit requires time and energy.

Over time, your thoughts can shift.

Positive self-talk can happen to be your norm.

The following under listed tips can assist you in how to practice self-talk:

> **Utilize your feelings to check-in.**

Stop during events or unpleasant days and check your self-talk.

Is it becoming negative? How can you transform it?

> **Discover the humor.**

Laughter can assist relieve stress and tension.

When you need a lift for positive self-talk, discover ways to laugh, like watching funny animal videos or a comedy.

➤ **Pinpoint negative self-talk traps.**

Some scenarios may increase your self-doubt and cause more negative self-talk.

Work events, for instance, could be particularly hard.

Pinpointing when you experience the most negative self-talk can assist you to anticipate and prepare.

➤ **Offer yourself positive affirmations.**

Sometimes, seeing positive words or inspiring images are often enough to redirect your thoughts.

Post small reminders in your office, in your home, and anywhere you spend quality time.

➤ **Have yourself surrounded by positive persons.**

Whether or not you notice it, you can absorb the outlook and emotions of the persons around you.

This comprises of negative and positive, so choose positive persons once you can.

The appropriate time to seek support

Positive self-talk can assist you to improve your outlook on life.

It also can have lasting positive health benefits, including improved well-being and a far better quality of life.

However, self-talk is a habit made over a lifetime.

If you tend to possess negative self-talk and err on the side of pessimism, you can practice how to change it.

It requires time and constant practice, but it is possible you develop uplifting positive self-talk.

If you discover you are not successful on your own, discuss it with a therapist.

Mental health experts can assist you with pinpoint sources of negative self-talk and learn to flip the switch.

Ask your health care provider for a referral to a therapist, or find out from a friend or family member for a suggestion.

Negative Affirmations We Repeat in Our Heads

Affirmations are positive statements that can be utilized to assist you to overcome negative, self-sabotaging thoughts.

Although at the onset they can feel a little bit hard; they possess the ability to reprogram your mind.

When you repeat them regularly and believe in them you can really start to make positive changes in all areas of your life.

A little bit like going to yoga or fitness class regularly, the more you indulge in it, the more change you experience physically.

Affirmations are similar, they are simply exercises for the mind and by repeating them frequently you will experience mental changes.

Many persons possess an ongoing battle with that bad, negative voice in their heads.

'I am not good enough ... I am not skinny enough ... I am not confident enough'.

This is something that could have sat deep into our conscious and unconscious minds from childhood, maybe it was due to the bully at school.

If a belief is deeply rooted in the unconscious mind then it can be really hard to override that thought and feeling with a generic affirmation.

That is the reason why it is so vital when you are choosing your affirmations that it is relevant and true to you.

The following tips work together to enable mental resilience and a relaxed, clear mind:

1. Identify & Separate yourself from Negative Thought Patterns

Negative thought patterns are repetitive, limiting thoughts.

They directly result in what we could refer to as 'negative' (unwanted or unpleasant) emotions such as fear, stress, anxiety, depression, unworthiness, shame, etc.

Once we learn to identify negative thought patterns as they happen, we can begin to step back from them.

This process of stepping back or separating yourself from thoughts is named 'cognitive defusion.'

In cognitive defusion, we learn to ascertain the thoughts in our head as simply that—just thoughts.

Not reality.

You see once we are fused with our thoughts (cognitive fusion) we tend to be very serious with them.

We believe them, We buy into them and we obey them. We play them out.

There is something that is vital for you to know; it is completely normal to possess negative thoughts!

It is part of our evolutionary history.

There is absolutely nothing wrong with you.

We all have minds that have evolved to be constantly on the lookout for problems and dangers, so most of us possess minds prone to have a lot of negative thoughts.

The problem is not that we possess negative thoughts.

The problem comes once we believe our thoughts are right.

When you are no longer entangled in thoughts they lose their grip on you and lose their power to produce unpleasant emotions.

Imagine you are lying in a bed in the morning, you look through the window and you discover that it is raining and once again the thought arises "what a dreadful day".

If you are not fused with the thought (you do not buy into it) then your experience would be this way.

You are watching the rain falling, then you also watch the thought (as simply a mental event) "what a dreadful day" arise and fall away just as the rain is falling...and since you do not take it seriously or believe in it, it brings no negativity, passes by easily and you are free to lay there relaxed and at ease, enjoying the noise of the rain on the roof.

As you can see, the capability to recognize unhelpful thinking and separate yourself from it is incredibly liberating.

It can change the standard of your entire day and indeed your entire life.

It is important to be able to recognize the sorts of unhelpful thinking styles that may arise, so here are other negative thinking patterns that are commonest.

Check them out below.

Anxious thoughts and worry

Worry is when the mind projects into an imagined future and conjures up scenes and thoughts about what could fail.

Here it usually creates 'what if' scenarios.

Sometimes it takes the shape of imagining or expecting that bad things will occur or that nothing pleasant will ever happen for you.

You would possibly be bordered about your health degenerating, your relationship going down the drain, your car malfunctioning or your career being ruined—even though nothing has actually happened at that moment.

You might pay attention to the shortage in your life and believe that nothing will ever recover for you.

Stress associated with your financial future, the welfare of your children or your partner leaving you fit into this category.

Constant Criticism and self-beating

The second pattern of negative thought is to constantly criticize and 'self improve' because you are not adequate yet.

You may be quite harsh on yourself, focusing in on each of your weaknesses and perceived flaws.

Likewise, you may extend this habit of criticism to other persons in your life.

This can be the result of tremendous strain on relationships.

Negative self-talk and self-criticism usually result in low self-esteem and a scarcity of confidence.

One way some persons deal with low self-esteem is to catch up on these feelings by attaining status, achievements, and recognition.

Others may feel completely debilitated by feelings of unworthiness, becoming depressed or maybe suicidal.

There is nothing bad with having goals and focusing to get fitter or healthier and therefore the like; we can simply prefer to do those because they are good for us or we would like to stretch and grow.

It is a really distinct headspace to be doing those things because we do not desire we are enough yet.

When the mind continuously hones in on what is bad with yourself (and your life) and disassociates from what is going well and is good, we will become stuck in negativity.

Constant guilt and regret

Ruminating on mistakes made within the past usually creates feelings of shame, guilt, and negativity.

Feelings of worthlessness may come up once you play over and over in your mind, 'bad' choices or 'wrong' actions you are feeling you have done.

There is nothing 'negative' per se' about simply reflecting on previous experiences.

This is usually how we will learn, grow and mature as individuals.

Negativity arises once you linger over a situation repeatedly with no real intention to learn and grow—but instead, you are self-beating or wishing things were different rather than being accepting of things as they are.

Problems

Negative thoughts usually revolve around what is not right with your life.

Your attention becomes fixated on and exaggerates the so-called negative aspects of your life.

Here your mind will usually downplay what is going well.

For instance, you may have an exquisite family, food to eat and shelter, but your car breaks down and it is all you can put your mind at and focus all week long.

You permit things with the car to dominate your thinking and negative emotions arise as a result.

All week you are frustrated, angry and depressed due to the car when your focus might be expanded to what is going well and what you are grateful for.

The reality is that the car is faulty.

It is not running any longer and needs to be taken to the mechanic workshop.

That is an easy fact.

Ruminating continuously on things is not constructive at all and is another means we will get trapped in negativity.

If you have got this habit of lamenting over your sorrows and problems you will constantly feel frustrated, depressed, anxious, and apathetic.

When you are so absorbed in what is wrong, you are not able to note what is good.

2. How to come to your senses

Notice that a lot of negative thoughts mostly flow from two different directions.

The first is dwelling on the past; maybe you ruminate over mistakes, problems, guilt and anything in your life that did not go the way you envisaged it should have gone.

The second is worrying about the future; fear of what may or may not occur for yourself, others or the world.

This may take the form of stress over whether or not you will achieve certain goals or anxiety about the safety of your finances or relationships.

Or perhaps you may worry about aging.

Whatever your particular negative thoughts are, notice that so as to interact in negative thought patterns the mind must cast its focus mostly into past or future.

Either that or we judge and mentally label things within the here and now to be 'unpleasant'.

When lost in negative thinking we tend to be so occupying in thoughts that we totally lose touch with what is actually going on in the present moments of our lives.

We miss the small pleasures of living every day.

The sunlight on your skin, the taste of the food we are eating, a real connection with somebody we love while they are talking.

When we are lost on our heads we lose touch with the planet around us, and we lose touch with ourselves.

To become more present, and capable of stepping out of negative thinking, one powerful method is to 'come to your senses'.

In order to do this simply redirect your attention out of the thoughts in your head and convey your focus to your sense perceptions.

Whether you are present in your home, at the office, within the park or on a subway, notice all the things around you.

Utilize your senses to their fullest.

Do not get into a mental dialogue about what you see, just be aware of what you are experiencing at that time.

Be aware of the sounds, the scents, and the sensation of the air on your skin or the contact points with the seat under you.

Be there fully in the moment.

This is a form of mindfulness practice

Now, it is not that we are aiming to live completely immersed in our senses at all times.

It is right to think when it is useful of course.

But we can utilize this awareness of our senses to the ground and center us in a greater awareness when we discover ourselves caught up in negative thinking.

It is actually almost not possible to be both deeply present at the moment in our senses and keep the negativity going.

Attempt it as an experiment and see for yourself if this is true.

3. Frequent mindfulness practice

Mindfulness is simply described as the practice of waking up to that wellspring of wholeness and peace.

It is waking up out of mind wandering (where we are lost in our heads, habits, our old beliefs, reactions, and thinking patterns) so that we are been able to live deliberately.

Through mindfulness, our capacity to live is been built from that deeper awareness and tame the mind.

Frequent mindfulness meditation has been indicated to decrease depression, stress and anxiety also as improving immune function.

There exists a lot of power in this simple practice.

By practicing daily mindfulness meditation you will gradually cultivate more awareness and be less trapped in your mind.

4. Ask helpful questions for unhelpful thoughts

Some sorts of negative thinking patterns are often quite 'sticky'.

You may discover that you try to 'name it to tame it' and come back to your senses but the thoughts continue to possess a grip on you.

If you find yourself in this situation there are some further tools you can utilize to untangle your thoughts and vary your focus.

These are referred to as helpful questions for unhelpful thoughts.

You can utilize a few of these questions to mentally question negative thoughts and utilize others to vary your focus.

Here are some questions you can ask yourself to assist you to untangle from the thought.

You ask them and then you can give an answer to them in your head.

Usually you would just pick one among these at any given duration.

- Is this thought useful or helpful in any way?
- Is it true? (Can I totally know that it is true)
- Is this simply an old story that my mind is playing out of habit?
- Does this thought assist me to take effective action?
- Is this though of great help or is my mind just babbling on?

Then you will (mentally) ask these questions below to make a recent focus and recent possibilities.

These questions will assist you to focus on constructive thoughts and actions and assist you effectively face your daily challenges and move towards living a more meaningful life.

Again, you may only use these at a time but you could usually try more than one too.

- What is the truth? My deepest truth?

- What do I actually want to feel or create in the situation?

- In what way can I move towards that?

- How can I produce the best in this situation?

- Who would I be in the absence of this negative thought?

- What recent story or thought can I focus on at this moment?

With these powerful questions, you can vary your focus from being stuck in negativity to being focused on what is going nicely.

They will as well assist you to take constructive action and move towards living a more meaningful life.

Constructive thinking permits you to be happy when things are going well and puts problems in perspective when times get tough so you will stay calm and clear-headed and deal with them in a practical efficient way.

Chapter 3

How to Use Positive Affirmations Effectively

Science has indicated that affirmations, when done appropriately, are an efficient tool for quickly becoming the person you desire to be to achieve everything you would like in your life.

Nonetheless, affirmations as well, possess a bad rap.

Many persons have tried them only to be disappointed, with little or no positive outcome.

The cause of the disappointment is that the ancient way of doing affirmations does not work.

For many years, myriads of experts and gurus have taught affirmations in ways in which have shown to be ineffective and set you up for failure, time and time again.

There exist two common problems with affirmations.

Firstly, lying to yourself does not work.

I am a millionaire; no you are not.

I have 7 percent body fat; no you do not.

I have achieved every one of my goals this year; no you have not.

This pattern of making affirmations that are written as if you have already become or achieved something could also be the only biggest reason that affirmations have not worked for many persons.

With this system, whenever you recite an affirmation that simply is not rooted in fact, your subconscious will resist it.

As an intelligent person who is not delusional, lying to yourself repeatedly can never be the optimum strategy.

The truth will always stand.

The second major reason for disappointment with affirmations is that passive language does not yield results.

Many affirmations are designed to enable you to feel good by creating an empty promise of something you want.

For instance, here is a common "money" affirmation that is been perpetuated for many years, by many world-famous gurus:

I am a money magnet. Money flows to me effortlessly and in abundance.

This type of affirmation might cause you to feel good within the moment by supplying you with a false sense of relief from your financial worries, but it will not generate any income.

Individuals who sit back and await the money to magically show up are cash poor.

To generate financial abundance (or any result you want, for that matter), you have to actually do something.

Your actions must be in alignment together with your desired results, and your affirmations must articulate and affirm both.

Affirmations can assist take your world from negative to positive in only a couple of minutes each day.

These little sayings are positive statements that can assist keep you motivated and develop a more positive perception of yourself.

Affirmations can not only assist you to change negative thoughts, but they can also as well motivate you to accomplish major goals.

Affirmations are simple to make and utilize, but you will require dedication to enable them to work.

How to optimize your positive affirmations

1. Utilize your affirmations as a map for change.

Affirmations are often a strong self-help tool, but just saying them is merely a part of the process.

Affirmations got to be including action so as to be truly effective.

Use your affirmation as a guide for the change you would like to cause in your life.

Then, take action to pursue that change.

> ➤ If you need that promotion, make an affirmation notifying yourself that you are worthy.
>
> Then, update your resume, put together a strong proposal, and let your boss be aware.
>
> Your affirmation will assist you to see that you are capable, and your actions will get the job done.

> ➤ Utilize your affirmation as a reminder of the fact that you can be the person you desire to be.
>
> It ought to highlight some of your best traits.
>
> Reflect on those when things don't go smoothly.

2. Write out your affirmations in addition to saying them.

In addition to saying your affirmations each day, write them out when you are less busy.

This offers distinct mental feedback than saying your affirmations, which may assist to further reinforce your goals and strengths.

It is also a good way to utilize your affirmation at places like work or school when you need it, but do not want others to hear it.

> ➤ You could make a decision that you want to write out your affirmation a given number of times, such as at least 10 times prior to your bedtime.
> ➤ Post your affirmations in areas where you will see them frequently.
>
>   Put one on your mirror, desk, car dashboard, or computer.
>
>   Slip one into your wallet or carry a little notebook with you.

> Alternatively, you may make a decision that you only want to write it out when you are feeling especially stressed or upset.

3. Do a meditation on your affirmations.

Close your eyes; breathe deeply, attempt to shut out the rest of the world and think about your affirmations.

Slowly and calmly repeat the words, thinking about what each one entails to you.

Visualize the positive feelings you desire to create or the goals you want to achieve every time you say your affirmation.

> If you are new to meditation, begin by taking a few slow, deep breaths and trying to clear your mind.
>
> You probably will not get all the noise out your first few times, and that is alright.
>
> The simple act of attempting can still possess positive effects.

Utilizing affirmations to combat negative thinking

1. Make a list of the negative thoughts you would like to get rid of.

Affirmations are useful in turning your negative thoughts into positives.

To effectively combat those thoughts, though, you would like to first identify them.

Begin by writing out a list of the negative thoughts you want to work on getting rid of utilizing positive affirmations.

> ➤ For instance, if you constantly tell yourself that you are ugly and worthless, two negative thoughts worth writing down would be, "I think I do not contribute to the world around me," and "I am not happy with my appearance."

> ➤ Write down a lot of negative thoughts as you feel comfortable bringing up. At this moment, you are just brainstorming things you may want to tackle.

2. Prioritize your list to pinpoint what you want to work on.

Once you are through with your list of negative thoughts, think about which ones impact you the most in your day to day life.

To get the most out of your affirmations, you will want to focus on one or two pieces of negative self-talk at a time.

Utilize your list to assist you to decide which negative thoughts you want to get rid of the most.

> It can be tempting to try to conquer each of your negative thoughts.

Ultimately, though, you will have more success if you begin with just one or two and work your way through.

> Try writing down whatever negative thoughts you have each day.

After a week or 2, look at this journal to see what sorts of concerns or criticisms you keep having.

These repeat thoughts should probably be a priority to fix.

3. Create your affirmation using your counter-argument.

Utilizing your counter-argument as guidance, write out your affirmation.

Your affirmation should identify yourself in a positive light and frame you as the sort of person you value.

It should as well utilize the emotions you identified in your counter-argument to support yourself and verify why you are worth your while.

> ➤ For instance, a college student that feels unintelligent may say, "I am an intelligent, capable student who is on their way to graduating."
>
> Someone struggling with depression may write, "I am a loving, caring person that deserves to be happy."

4. Repeat your affirmation each day for at least 5 minutes.

Take at least 5 minutes each day to say your affirmation to yourself over and over.

If you can, check out yourself directly in the mirror and say your affirmation aloud during this point.

It is going to feel uncomfortable at the beginning, but affirmations only work through repetition.

Sometimes you just have to put on a "fake it 'till you make it" mentality.

➢ Continue this process for as long as you want to counteract your negative thought.

For some persons, this may be a matter of several weeks.

For others, it could take months or maybe years.

➢ Your affirmation will gradually force your brain to confront the disconnect between what you are saying and how you view yourself.

Repeating your affirmation assists retrain your brain to stop feeling so uncomfortable when you think positively about yourself.

Visualizing positive results with affirmations

1. Write out your positive attributes.

We hardly focus on what we like about ourselves, but our strengths are hugely vital in accomplishing our goals.

An inventory of your positive traits will assist you to see all your personal strengths.

Write down a list of all your positive attributes to assist guide your affirmation.

> ➢ Take stock of yourself by making a list of your best qualities, capabilities, or other attributes: Are you gorgeous? Write it down. Are you a hard worker? Make note of it.

> ➢ Make your sentences short, first-person statements such as "I am generous," for instance, or "I can speak 4 languages."

> ➢ If you are struggling to think of positive things, challenge yourself to write at least 5 positives to begin.

You may find that once you get going, you are more comfortable with the activity.

> Try finding out from someone for their opinion on what your positive attributes are.

They may identify characteristics that you have not observed about yourself.

2. Have your desired goal or outcome set.

Your affirmation will work more effectively when it targets a specific goal or outcome.

Your goal may be ongoing, such as being more confident or getting ahead in your career.

It could as well have a set deadline, such as finishing a project on time or being ready for a big event.

> Picking an outcome will assist you to target your affirmation and give it real applications in your day to day life.

> Give yourself adequate time to reach your goal or to develop a new habit.

It can take around 66 days to form a new habit or to change an existing one.

3. Say your affirmation each day for at least 5 minutes.

For your affirmation to work effectively, you need to expose yourself to it each passing day.

Stand in front of the mirror and say your affirmation out loud over and over again for at least minutes.

The more you say your affirmation, the more you are encouraging your brain to visualize your positive outcome.

> ➢ If you can take 5 minutes twice each day to say your affirmation, that is even better.

4. Match up some of your positive attributes with your goals.

Ask yourself which of your positive qualities will assist you to achieve the goals or reach the outcome you desire.

If you are quitting smoking, for instance, you may draw upon your willpower or courage.

If you are trying to pass a class, you may want to focus more on your intelligence and determination.

Your affirmations ought to be posted in important places.

Male use of sticky notes, cards, a cute poster or printout, or any other system you like to write out your affirmation.

Leave these notes in places where it will not only be visible but need to be reminded of your affirmation.

Try to think of places where you regularly experience stress or self-doubt and put a copy of your affirmation there.

> ➤ Slip one inside your desk drawer, or stick one to your computer monitor.
>
> Put one up on the bathroom mirror, and stick one on the refrigerator.
>
> Every time you see the card, read it and think about what it entails to you.

> ➤ Carry your affirmation with you, too.
> Put a copy of your affirmation inside your wallet or purse.

If you need a pick-me-up, or if you find yourself about to waver from your goals, bring it out and repeat it to yourself.

List Of Affirmation Applications You Can Use

For most folks, calling up positive phrases and pictures on a constant basis is not easy; not only can we need to wrestle with the negative thoughts and experiences that surround us, we even have to create time to re-center our thoughts.

That is the reason the under listed apps exist.

Each of them possesses the power to make you feel good about yourself no matter where you are or what you're doing.

Give these apps a try if you would like to incorporate more positive affirmations in your daily life:

1. Shine

Shine is simply a text messaging service based on the thought that sometimes, you would like some external phrases to guide your internal positive thinking.

Visit the website, and you will have the ability to sign up to receive a daily text message; all you need to provide is a first name and a phone number.

Then, Monday through Friday, you will receive one message per day with inspirational quotes from successful individuals, links to research-backed articles you will utilize as motivation, and recommendations on actions you can take to feel more positive in your day to day life.

2. Smiling Mind

Smiling Mind is described as a nonprofit organization that is attempting to make a positive experience of mindfulness meditation available for everyone.

Because the organization was founded by and is currently operated by psychologists and educators, every operation they do is backed by scientific evidence, so you can ensure your new habits and affirmations are guiding you in the proper direction.

In the app, you will discover a variety of various guided meditation options, which may assist you to eliminate your negative thoughts and pay attention to the positivity of these moments.

There are distinct programs for distinct age groups including children as young as 7 years old to adults, and programs for specific applications, such as meditation for education, sports, and the workplace.

You can as well track your progress since the app records how long your sessions are and the time you have participated in those sessions.

The app is free to use but you will make a donation if you would like to continue supporting their efforts.

The app is out there for Apple and Android devices.

3. Grateful

Gratitude journals are a well-known way to practice positive affirmations since they force you to slow down and focus on the positive things that are already present in your life.

Then, once recorded, you can go back and look at positive experiences in the past for inspiration.

Now, you can utilize an app to make the process of gratitude journaling simpler and more enjoyable; not to mention more consistent.

Grateful is an app that offers you daily prompts; every day, you will be met with a question like "what made you smile today" or "why was today a good day?"

Answering with even one word is often a positive affirmation in its title but the app permits you to write down the maximum amount as you would like or maybe add a photo.

4. Happify

No matter what your goals are for establishing more positivity and better emotional wellbeing in your life, Happify has something which will assist you.

In the world of their own, "Happify happens to be the single destination for effective, evidence-based solutions for better emotional health and wellbeing within the 21st century."

The major perk here is that the app assists you measure your subjective feelings of happiness over the course of weeks and months, so you will see the patterns in your emotions and (hopefully) notice a pattern of improvement.

While using the app, you will discover tools designed to break up negative thoughts, reduce your stress, and build confidence, including positive affirmations and activities meant to assist you relax.

You will even discover guided meditation sessions, helping you create the foremost of this moment, wherever you are.

5. ThinkUp

Once you download the app, you will be capable to begin recording your own positive affirmations in your own voice.

If you are feeling confident and good about your place in life, you will come up with some positive statements about yourself and have them recorded for posterity.

If you are feeling less creative or do not know what to mention, do not worry—the app also features a list of generic positive statements that you simply can peruse and choose between.

Once you've got a variety of recorded phrases, you will begin taking note of them however you would like; for instance, you will have them randomly mixed into the music you are listening to, or set a schedule so you hear your affirmations at regular intervals.

6. Kwippy

Positivity can surface in a lot of forms.

In many cases, affirmations that come from others are often more powerful than ones you utter to yourself.

That is where Kwippy comes in.

Kwippy is a new sort of social media platform which will send you random challenges throughout the day, prompting you to snap a photograph of something in your nearby environment.

For instance, a challenge could be "take a selfie with the closest living thing."

Users can view photo submissions from every other user (as all Kwippy users receive an equivalent challenge at the same time), and are given an opportunity to vote on the photos they think best capture the theme (or those that are the foremost entertaining).

You will also be able to comment on other images.

If you are having an unpleasant day, the prompts are often your chance to re-center yourself and be mindful of this moment, and therefore the affirmations from people once they see your contribution are often precisely the motivation you would like to keep going.

7. Bmindful

Bmindful does not have the fancy interface that a lot of the apps on this list do, and it exists solely as a web app.

But while it lacks in design or mobile functionality, it makes up for with a huge and ever-growing list of affirmations you will utilize to introduce more positivity into your life.

Once you sign up for free of charge, you will possess the power to create an inventory of your own personal affirmations, curated from massive topic-based lists written by the community.

Categories comprise things such as health, love, life, success, wealth, money, relationships, abundance, confidence, work, strength and creativity.

You can have them organize the way you see fit, and write your own affirmations—either for your private use or to share with other community members.

Soon, you will have a huge list of affirmations that make sense to you, and specifically, you can turn to that list whenever you require a break from your negative thoughts.

8. Instar Affirmation Writer

Instar Affirmation Writer is an app for individuals that want to take charge of writing and managing their own affirmations, instead of counting on those written by other individuals.

Within the app, you will have the power to schedule alerts and reminders for yourself, so you write new positive affirmations on a frequent basis and therefore the app will notify you when it detects key criteria being met in your response, including focusing on the recent moment and an entire "positive" emotion.

You can have your own voice recorded reading these affirmations, and enhance the affirmations you write with ongoing tips.

On top of that, you will categorize all of your affirmations and concentrate on how often you affirm by monitoring your writing patterns.

The app is available on the App Store.

Chapter 4

Common Challenges on Using Affirmations

In your entire life, you have been hearing about positive affirmations and therefore the power of positive thinking.

Maybe you have even posted phrases all over your apartment; for instance, phrases such as "I am super-rich." or "I attract only positive people into my life."

On the other hand, when you move around your apartment and realize you are having trouble paying the rent and your boss at work is anything but positive, that gap leads to even more frustration, guilt, and feelings of failure.

You try to remain positive, to believe it is coming "one day", but in the meantime, your life feels stuck and out of touch with your beliefs.

The following are common challenges of using affirmations:

Your beliefs will not allow you to be wrong.

Your subconscious beliefs, the stories you have developed about the person you are, and therefore the unique perspectives that you simply have held all of your life are what really rule your reality.

In fact, your subconscious will do just about anything to ensure what you believe is validated to you in the world.

It is a mechanism we have for staying sane, but it can as well work against us.

For instance, if you think that life is a struggle, that in your family nobody was fortunate or that everybody but you seems to achieve success, then you will read an affirmation a day about getting rich and your subconscious reacts with it.

You are been disconnected from your original Self.

Sometimes you think that you want something that is actually incongruent with what you truly desire.

You think you would like to be rich or famous, but at heart, your Authentic Spirit is far more curious about freedom of time or meaningful relationships or an easy life.

When your personal values conflict with what you are requesting for, your actual life choices could be reflecting something different than your affirmation.

You based your positive affirmations outside of yourself.

An affirmation must be about you, not about the planet out there.

You only have control over yourself.

You can change your own beliefs, your own behaviors, your own perspective about what occurs then, in turn, this may be reflected by your external reality.

The Best Way to Recite Affirmations

It is ideal we recite affirmations the right way in order for them to work effectively for us.

The following are what you will do to ensure they work for you to assist you to achieve your goals and maximize your potential within your most vital roles.

1. Set a reminder

Set a reminder in your calendar, not exceeding monthly intervals and not below annual intervals, to review your affirmations and for everyone to ask the question "How has this affirmation changed my behavior in a tangible way since the review?"

If you cannot consider a true result you have achieved from the affirmation make a goal associated with it alongside action steps to realize that goal.

This will give your affirmation the weight of action and you will find it more meaningful when you have it repeated.

2. Always be sincere

One interesting thing about sincerity is that you can trick yourself into it by wanting to want what you should want.

If I feel insincere saying "I eat healthful foods" or even "I want to eat healthful foods" I can say "I want to want to eat healthful foods."

I have utilized this trick time and time again and it works for me, that is, it changes how I feel and results in positive changes in behavior that produce the outcomes I desire.

3. Do not attempt to do too much

People who are walking around as perfectionists are ultimately scared that the world is going to view them for who they actually are.

Perfectionism is negative behavior.

First, it represents a false reality that we will become perfect.

Second, when we fail, it tells us that we are hopeless failures.

The end results are anxiety, paralysis, stress, guilt, and limited potential.

4. Have a solid plan

If you fail to plan you plan to fail.

The point of affirmations is not that they are doing all the work for you, instead, they assist you to modify your behavior to obtain better results.

Affirmations ought to be accompanied by goals, plans, programs, schedules, and other tools that will assist make those affirmations reality.

Recite Affirmations in Front of a Mirror and Why it is Very Powerful

I love mirrors.

I love them due to the fact that they assist us to learn things about ourselves and they possess the power to change the inside by looking at the outside.

What we tell ourselves in front of the mirror possess a good effect on what we say to ourselves internally.

Our thoughts are affirmations we tell ourselves within the inside and they can direct us towards a cheerful life or painful life.

If we are saying goodies to ourselves, we will focus on the good and our life will improve.

If we are saying bad things, we will focus on heartache and pain and obtain more of them in our life.

The following are unique daily affirmations you should say to yourself in front of the mirror every morning.

Sometimes, you just need a reminder.

It sure, it is cheaper and shorter than taking some drugs or going to a therapist.

- I am pretty
- I am special
- I respect myself
- I am kind
- I am sexy
- I am proud of myself
- I am valuable and worthy
- I am OK
- I am enough
- I can do it
- I love my body
- I am free
- I am safe
- I am grateful
- Every breath I take is a new beginning.
- I am perfect the way I am
- I am strong
- With the body I have, I can experience joy and happiness.
- If my mind is telling me bad things about me, I don't have to listen
- I see good everywhere
- Everything will be OK in the end. If it's not OK, it's not the end

Chapter 5

"I AM" the Powerful Affirmation

Affirmations are very powerful.

Your subconscious mind does not function in terms of past, present or future.

If you affirm that you "want" something, then you get "the wanting" but you do not actually get the thing that you are wanting.

The words "I am" are two of the most powerful words in human languages.

It does not matter the dialect or culture.

Whatever you put behind these words automatically become your reality.

In order to get what you would like, affirmations must be at the present tense.

When you say I am HAPPINESS, then life will provide you the means to.

Human beings possess two main powers on Earth: Awareness and Choice.

Become aware of who you really are so that you can make a good choice.

You are a blessing.

You are unique.

You are a gift to the whole world.

Learn positive words in order for you to become conscious of who you really are.

You are magnificent.

You are Love.

You are Pure Love and Light.

Affirm it!

Below is a huge list of affirmations that begin with "I AM"

- ➤ I am special.
- ➤ I am at ease with the uncontrollable things occurring in my life. I am prepared for any challenges.
- ➤ I am aware of my mistakes and I learned from them.
- ➤ I am calm and relaxed in every circumstance.

- I am the creator of my personal life. I build its foundation and that I choose its content.
- I am filled with strength and I exude happiness.
- I am loyal I am at peace with myself.
- I am open-minded and that I fully take advantage of all opportunities surrounding me.
- I am able to do amazing things.
- I am worthy.
- I am balanced.
- I am more than enough.
- I am full-hearted.
- I am very superior to negative thoughts and low actions.
- I am blessed with infinite talents and I make use of them every single day.
- I am at peace with everything that occurred.
- I am a wonderful human being.
- I am proud of all the things that I have accomplished so far.

- I am ambitious.
- I am fearless and I take risks.
- I am curious.
- I am a learner.
- I am grateful for my life.
- I am inspired by recent and good ideas.
- I am content with each of my accomplishments.
- I am brave and I am kind.
- I am a positive person and my entire life is crammed with prosperity.
- I am admired and lots of persons acknowledge my results.
- I am blessed with health and motivation.
- I am indestructible.
- I am always happy around other persons.
- I am capable to achieve great things in my life. I am comfortable being alone in my very own company.
- I am positive.
- I am productive.

- I am on top of everything in my life.
- I am a hard worker.
- I am respected.
- I am filled with energy and determination.
- I am aware of my value and I never allow others to bring me down.
- I am free to be myself.
- I am productive motivated and extremely hardworking.
- I am worthy of abundance in all things that I do.
- I am a creator.
- I am important.
- I am worthy to be loved and respected by a wonderful partner.
- I am safe in the world and life loves and supports me.
- I am ready to change.
- I am providing for my body with solely healthy foods my body is my protection.
- I am on an ever-changing journey.
- I am grateful for my healthy body. I love life.

- I am cleaned by negative thoughts or bad habits.
- I am a strong person I face fear with power and kindness.
- I am in charge. I now take my own power back.
- I am aware that each day may be a sacred gift from life.
- I am strong enough to live my dreams. I release all negative thoughts of the past and every worry concerning the future.
- I am loved; love flows through my whole body and it releases any disease affecting it.
- I am constantly willing to find out there is always room for more.
- I am becoming better and better each day.
- I am in love with all that I am and I accept that which I cannot control.
- I am loved and prosperous every single day.
- I am as special as anyone else living in this world.
- I am well educated.
- I am patient.

- I am a fighter.
- I am responsible for how I feel and I always choose happiness.
- I am my personal superhero.
- I am choosing and not waiting to be the one to be chosen.

How Often To Recite Affirmations

Your mind happens to be the most receptive first thing in the morning after you rise and also right before you fall asleep, so those two times of the day are very vital.

The third time should be a time of day once you can focus on your affirmation and reflect thereon for just a moment or two without distractions.

You do not need a lot of time, the important factor here is that you do not just say the affirmation, but feel it as well.
Mixing your affirmations with emotion is where the vital magic is in reciting affirmations, so ensure you give yourself that moment to actually feel what you are saying to yourself.

A lot of affirmation practitioners claim that daily affirmations ought to be repeated a specific number of times, but I disagree.

Being obsessed with an exact number of repetitions is highly distracting and counterproductive.

Rather than repeating a precise number of times, it is ideal you set a timer for 5 or 10 minutes (depending on how much free time you have) and slowly repeat your affirmations with conviction until the timer goes off.

This permits you to focus on your affirmations and pause between them rather than worry about counting to 500 or 1,000 or whatever.

People that suggested affirmations ought to be recited multiple times a day mean well and the advice somewhat rooted in logic.

After all, the logic behind this advice is solid on the conscious level, but it is not your conscious mind that needs to be reached – it is your subconscious mind.

Your conscious mind and the thousand repetitions per day only assist in the respect that it can help you build the habit of repeating your affirmations and force you to do it once you do not desire it.

No doubt, making affirmations a daily habit is vital and a certain amount of repetition is necessary to reinforce habits, but reaching your mind on a subconscious level is far more vital.

The way the mind-body connection reduces affirmation repetitions

Realistically, who is going to spend more than 5 or 10 minutes at a go reciting affirmations?

Certainly nobody.

It is not engaging or appealing, and therefore, will not assist to build a daily affirmation habit.

If you want to be efficient and reduce the amount of time spent on your affirmations, think about how you deliver your affirmations to yourself.

You have to involve your whole body in the process – not only your brain.
To reduce the number of times I need to repeat my affirmations every day also as to reduce the overall time I spend on a particular affirmation theme (self-esteem, finance, etc.), I include movement into my daily routine.

Specifically, I have my affirmations repeated in front of a mirror or sometimes I just do it while standing up if I do not have access to any mirror.

I have never recited my affirmations while sitting down because it does not have a similar powerful effect.

Based on some years of experience manifesting my desires and affirming my way out of unhealthy beliefs, I have discovered that I need to be pacing, standing, or at the very least moving my hands around and looking myself in the eye in a mirror in order for my affirmations to sink in and begin manifesting.

Otherwise, I could spend months on the same affirmations and make zero success.

I strongly believe that this all has something to do with the fact that movement is beneficial to learning.

After all, are we not repeating affirmations as a way to learn (or re-learn) how to do, have, be, believe, or act a particular way?

So as to plant the seed of improvement in our subconscious, we ought to make a genuine connection and feel it throughout the entire body. The body and mind are connected actually.

Chapter 6

Forms of Affirmations

Verbal Affirmations

Affirmations are words that simply uplift your thoughts.

By getting rid of negative thoughts and speaking in a confident way, you permit the creation and manifestation of all things positive and optimistic.

When you speak positive affirmations aloud, you are having your mind rewired to believe that your words are universal truths.

You at the same time raise the "feel-good levels" in your body, causing your brain to make recent neural networks that aid positive thinking.

Verbal affirmations offer you the courage to believe in yourself, enhance your entire well-being, and cultivate a deeper sense of self-love.

In life, there is just one relationship that you have to consistently maintain – and it is with yourself.

Appreciating and accepting yourself offers you the power to be anything you can desire being.

It assists you to become more influential in your own life, and assists you remain in the right frame of mind to assist you to reach your goals.

Written Statement

Want to understand the way to write affirmations that basically work?

The following easy tips will assist you to create affirmations that are extremely powerful and effective.

There are a few vital do's and don'ts when it comes to writing affirmations for yourself, so take a moment to review these step by step instructions and you will be capable to write positive affirmations that are supercharged in no time at all.

Getting Started

The simplest way to begin writing affirmations is to write down a list of "I am" statements that describe what you would like to possess or experience.

"I am happy"

"I am wealthy"

Notice that we did not use the phrase "I want" in any of these affirmations.

There is a vital reason for this.

If you start any affirmations with phrases like "I want" or "I need" then what you are affirming to yourself is the feeling of wanting and/or needing.

Rather, you ought to aim to affirm the sensation of already having what you desire.

Close your eyes and visualize that you are already going through the wonderful things that you desire, and write down your affirmations as an expression of "grateful having", instead of wanting or needing.

Here is just a single example:

"I am so excited and thankful for my wonderful new house"

You can also start your affirmations with words like:

"I know..."

"I have..."

"I love..."

or any other positive, affirmative statement.

Write down your affirmations in the positive

Write down your affirmations in such a way that they concentrate on what you would like, instead of what you are trying to avoid or get rid of from your life.

For instance, instead of writing "I am not hooked into cigarettes", a far better choice would be something like, "I am completely free from cigarettes".

In the second instance, we have removed the word "hooked in" and replaced it with the word "free".

Here is another example: Rather than writing "I am getting out of debt now", a more positive choice would be "I am wealthy and prosperous".

Notice the difference?

If you are feeling uncertain about the way to write affirmations in the positive, then imagine that you have already accomplished whatever it is that you wish to realize, then describe yourself in that positive light.

If you discover yourself starting an affirmation with the words "I am not..." please take pause and consider a more positive way to express yourself.

Write your affirmations in now

When you write down your affirmations, write them in the present.

Write as if you are experiencing what you desire immediately.

Do not make use of words such as, "Within the next two months...".

Why?

Because each time you utilize this affirmation, you are saying that you still have up to two months away from achieving your goal!

After one month of using this affirmation, you will still be saying "within two months..."

Utilize your affirmations to make an inner experience of getting what you desire immediately.

"I am healing"

"I am a wonderful and gifted artist"

Do you notice that these two example affirmations make no reference to dates or times?

They are simple, powerful affirmations of already possessing.

Always be yourself

Make use of words and phrases that are typical of your own way of thinking and speaking.

You are not writing affirmations for somebody else's benefit, you are writing affirmations for your own self...so be yourself!

You can be as silly or as serious or as plain or as colorful as you wish ...just be you!

Write your affirmations with so much passion and feelings

Think about how good you will feel once you achieve your goals, and how good it feels to know that positive changes are happening.

Include affirmations that describe these positive feelings of success.

For instance, if you have just written, "I am experiencing great success in my business", you might like to follow it up with something such as, "I am so excited to be enjoying all this wealth at last".

If you have written, "I am a very creative genius and I am always discovering amazing new ideas", you would possibly wish to add, "I feel so grateful for all the inspiration that comes to me".

If you would like to understand the way to write affirmations that are really effective, bear this in mind.

When you give a description of your feelings of affirmations, you connect with them more deeply.

Your affirmations will even have more power if you experience them on both a thinking and a sensible level.

Listening to music while you recite your affirmations can be of great benefit.

Music assists to engage your emotions, so that you are more able to tap into the feeling of what you wish to affirm.

Try listening to some inspirational music or some relaxing music...whatever assists to get you "in the zone".

Avoid not to get caught up in the "how"

If you are setting goals in your life, it is usually a great idea to have an action plan.

However, you ought not to create affirmations that describe all the small print about HOW you are going to achieve your goals.

Be as specific as you like about what you want to manifest with your affirmations, but do not try to define how these things will show up.

All you are required to do is put yourself in the frame of mind of already having what you would like, then let the universe find out the foremost efficient and harmonious way to bring it to you.

It may or may not come through the plan you had in mind.

Affirm your present successes as well

Your affirmations do not all have to be concerning things that you want or that are currently absent from your life.

Consider your positive attributes and therefore the things that are already working well for you.

Think about the things you admire about yourself and therefore the things that you simply are already grateful for.

Include some of these in your affirmations also.

So often we jettison to give ourselves credit for the things that we like about ourselves, so when writing affirmations, feel free to describe some of the things that you already appreciate about yourself and your life.

By so doing you will reinforce your positive feelings about who you are today, and you will be more open to accepting affirmations that describe who you desire to become.

Silent Repeat Thoughts

When these empowering statements are repeated all the time, they get into your subconscious and shut the doubting voices up.

You begin to notice yourself manifesting your goals and truly living your dreams. Confidence and faith generate greater motivation.

And when those 2 combined, you have got the results.

That is what is been referred to as "visualize, and realize".

Using affirmations is not only by reciting every day and wait for them to work.

If it is not appropriate for you to mention them aloud, repeat them to yourself mentally for an equivalent 3 times each day.

Engage your "mind muscles" while having them repeated in your head.

It almost seems like you are saying them aloud with all the muscles in your brain.

Audio Recordings

If you would like the very best in affirmation tapes, you ought to consider making your own.

Not only is it cheaper but, they may be far more effective than the commercial products on the market.

Virtually all research into accelerated learning has indicated that the more of your senses that you can involve in the process, the greater the effect you will possess on the learning process.

In developing your personal affirmation audios, you mix research and reading, writing, verbalizing and listening all at an equivalent time.

This enables your affirmations much more powerful.

In addition, you get to select the specific affirmations that will suit your needs.

While there are many excellent commercial audios available, they are designed for a wide audience.

If you make your own affirmation audios, you get to tailor the affirmations that will work more effectively for you.

Another reason to form your own audios is that they are going to be in your own voice.

Scientific research has indicated that the conscious and subconscious minds are far more sensitive to hearing your own voice.

So your mind is far more likely to implement your affirmations when they are in your own voice.

Create Your Own Positive Affirmations

Your outer world is a reflection of whatever is occurring in your inner world.

And, everything you experience stems from the quality of your thoughts and the belief you have about yourself.

Even though we throw the term "affirmations" around a lot and talk about how important they are, there seems to be some confusion around what they are and what makes them so powerful.

I can tell you from personal experience that putting daily affirmations into use in my life resulted in enormous results both personally and financially.

By utilizing the rules found below, you will be able to create your own positive affirmation effectively and experience an enormous change in your life.

1. Always be concise

Shorter is better.

Affirmations with lesser words are often easier to recall, especially in situations once you experience some stress.

Rhyming enables your affirmations even more memorable.

For instance, "I am feeling alive at 175."

2. Add action

Whenever possible, affirm yourself as an individual who takes action.

For instance: "I am thankfully driving my recent Rolls Royce along an open highway."

Action engages the Law of Attraction, creating recent results in our lives and unveiling us to further inspiration.

3. Say it in the present tense

Begin your affirmation by entering the present tense.

Take the condition you wish for and declare it to be true already.

4. Be positive

Our subconscious mind skips the word not.

So, remove this word from your affirmations.

"I am not scared of public speaking" gives us the message that you simply are scared.

Make use of, "I feel comfortable as I speak publicly."

5. Add a feeling word

Powerful affirmations comprise of content and emotion.

Content describes the specific outcome that you desire.

Emotion gets to the hearts of how you are feeling concerning that outcome.

For a more potent affirmation, add both elements.

Chapter 7:

List of 30 Categories of Positive Affirmations

1 – Health Affirmations

Health is wealth and positive health affirmations are the secret to wealth.

When the mind thinks health thoughts, the body finds it less difficult to be healthy.

The link between mind and body is now well identified.

It is an agreed incontrovertible fact that diseases are psychosomatic, i.e. they mostly occur by thought and emotions.

Even diseases caused by germs can be termed psychosomatic in the sense that germs are permitted to enter into the body or existing germs in the body become strong enough to result in the disease because the immune system of the body is lowered due to emotional reasons.

Emotions are been controlled by thought and thoughts can be formed at will.

Affirmations assist to mold thoughts.

Thus, the link between health affirmations and health becomes explicit.

It is possible to fill the mind with healthy thoughts by utilizing positive health affirmations.

Repeating these affirmations often impresses the subconscious to such a degree that it gradually begins transforming the body to align with the health thoughts.

Even dreaded diseases such as cancer are conquered by thought power.

The following are health affirmations that work magic:

- ➢ I nourish my mind, body, and soul each day.
- ➢ I choose health and wellbeing because I am worth it.
- ➢ My body is in perfect shape.
- ➢ My body is sturdy and healing.
- ➢ My body is fit and strong.
- ➢ My mind is calm and relaxed.
- ➢ My immune system is healthy and strong.
- ➢ My mind and body are healthy and very vibrant.
- ➢ I radiate confidence, health, and joy.

- My immune system is healing my body.
- My health is getting better every day.
- I am been surrounded by healing energy.
- I respect my body.
- My body is my vessel.
- I only put healthy foods inside my body.
- My body is strong and resilient.
- I am healed.
- I am healthy and whole.
- I have good health.
- I am grateful for my body.
- My body is gorgeous just the way it is.
- I love myself and my body.
- I choose good health for my whole life.
- I take good care of my body.
- I embrace the wisdom of my body.
- I am confident and comfortable with my body.
- I am grateful for my body's power and strength.
- I am aging gracefully.

- I look and feel youthful.

- I am grateful for good health at every age.

2 – Wellness Affirmations

Our thoughts and words that we repeat frequently possess the power to influence our minds and body.

Positive thoughts and positive words have the power to make and keep us healthy, and happier.

Naturally, we should always make it a habit to think twice before we speak.

In other words, our words have the power to build as well as to destroy.

Therefore, saying positive affirmations for well being could be a conscious effort to keep ourselves excited, energetic in life and luxuriate in healthiness and good relationship.

The following are affirmations for well being:

> ➤ I am blessed with abundant health

> ➤ I am blessed with perpetual well-being

> ➤ I am blessed with strength and wholeness

> ➤ I feel so special

- The universe is not a hostile place
- I am in the process of healing
- I claim health and peace for myself now
- My body is healthy and my mind is peaceful
- My whole thoughts are of abundant health and well-being
- I choose to feel good right now
- I love everything about myself
- I fully trust in the process of life
- I am healthy
- I am important
- I am happy and grateful
- I have unlimited potential
- I love my life
- I am relaxed, calm, and centered
- I am deserving of all good things
- I cherish this day this moment right now
- I am simply wonderful
- I choose to use positive uplifting self-talk
- I now prioritize for my well being

- I eat healthy food that nourishes my body
- I choose to enjoy myself and make life a playful experience
- I am powerful beyond my wildest dreams
- I create my reality
- I am passionate
- I focus on what is good concerning my life

3 – Healing Affirmations

Whatever our mind says influences our reality and creates the life we live this day.

Our minds and bodies work side by side in such a way that any thought we possess; whether it is positive or negative – reflects in the way we feel and look.

So if we want to have a more positive, happy life we need to align ourselves with the frequencies of happiness, joy, love, and gratitude.

We have to find ways to think about higher energy thoughts and avoid negative emotions, feelings, and thoughts as much as possible.

This is where affirmations for healing come into play.

When we repeat affirmations for healing with deep focus over and over again, they are carried into our subconscious mind and can change us on the levels of the mind over which we possess little to no conscious control over.

It is correct, we are what we think, but we have to bear in mind that we are far more than what we consciously think.

That is the reason it is detrimental to program our subconscious mind with positivity, joy, happiness, and healing so that we possess the power to manifest a life in harmony.

The following are a list of health affirmations that work very effectively.

> I am quitting all negative feelings

> I am strong, independent and respect my boundaries a lot

> I am quitting all negative feelings

> I am ready to be healed, so I permit forgiveness to manifest

> I believe in my capability to manifest happiness and healing

> I permit myself the time and space to heal

> I accept every emotion as guidance towards my healing

> I am surrounded by a person who loves me and who I really love

- ➤ I view every situation as a chance to heal and grow
- ➤ I am the master of my world. I release hurt. I enter the future with joy and enthusiasm.
- ➤ My body is getting stronger each day
- ➤ My body is healing itself
- ➤ Health is interested in me
- ➤ I have a robust body
- ➤ Each cell in my body vibrates energy and health
- ➤ I love and appreciate my body
- ➤ I am taking excellent care of myself
- ➤ I am blessed healthiness
- ➤ I am healed
- ➤ I look out for my body by making smart choices
- ➤ I am living in an extended and healthy life
- ➤ I vibrate health all over my body, mind, and soul
- ➤ My body deserves to be whole and healthy
- ➤ I choose happiness and health
- ➤ My body possesses a natural ability to heal.
- ➤ I am blessed with healthiness.

➢ My body is getting stronger each day.

➢ My body is healing by itself.

➢ The universe is blessing me with healthiness.

➢ I choose to be healthy, happy and whole.

4 – Self Care Affirmations

Have you ever tried saying self-care affirmations or mantras to urge you to think straight?

To assist you to gain a little control when feeling overwhelmed?

I strongly believe that they are very effective in helping you transform how you see and consider yourself.

And simply by practicing saying them frequently, you will be able to build a positive mental habit and a positive mindset.

They are truly essential in assisting you to condition your mind to assist you to gain a more positive outlook on life.

The following are a list of self-care affirmations:

➤ Each day, I choose to find out more about my authentic self.

➤ I am freed of self-doubt and self-sabotage.

➤ I am in total control of my negative thoughts.

➤ I choose to not take things personally.

➤ My daily commitment to my self-care is not selfish.

➤ I choose to abandon negative mental self-chatter.

➤ I am strong, empowered and capable of anything.

- I am deserving of all the great things in my life.
- I am very unique and nobody can ever do it exactly like me.
- My self-care is worth making time for.
- I am smart, courageous and self-confident.
- I am patient and good with myself and my progress.
- I am an independent thinker, not a nation pleaser.
- I am a top priority in my life.
- I have every right to mention no to anything that makes me feel uncomfortable.
- I must ensure I am regularly taking care of myself before I take on an excessive amount to assist others.
- I am liberated from expectations and criticism.
- I choose to forgive myself and abandoning of my past mistakes.
- I set healthy boundaries and take additional time to heal if needed.
- I honor my intuition and make use of it as a guide.
- I am liberated from other's negative vibes.

- ➤ I choose to abandon what I cannot control in my life.

- ➤ I choose to live within the moment.

- ➤ I nurture my creative side, the maximum amount as my practical side.

5 – Loving Yourself Affirmations

Self-love can be described as something we do not get enough of.

We are usually our own worst critics.

It is easy to be critical of our personal mistakes.

And that we could also be unforgiving once we fail.

If you desire to achieve success in life, it is very pertinent you love yourself.

People who want more than anything to find love got to love themselves first.

"Love thyself" is a few of the easiest advice ever written.

If you wish to do perfectly in just about anything, you need to love yourself.

Positive affirmations are an excellent way to bolster a flagging of self-love.

They are going to build your confidence in your best asset: yourself.

The following are affirmations for self-love:

- I feel profound empathy and love for other persons and their own unique paths.
- I choose to prevent apologizing for being me.
- I am at peace with everything that went on in my life.
- My entire life is crammed with joy and abundance.
- Happiness flows from me
- Positivity is a decision that I choose to make.
- I do not need other persons for happiness.
- I choose hope over fear.
- This day, I select me.
- I am deserving of infinite compassion.
- I will not take another person's negativity personally.
- I am ready to keep going, when things get tough, to realize the success I deserve
- My body is so gorgeous and expresses my spirit.
- I am grounded, peaceful, and centered.
- I respect my limitations and thank myself for the things I am prepared to accomplish.
- My commitment to myself is very real.

- I do not need others for happiness.
- I choose hope over fear.
- I am a diamond. It is the right time for me to shine.
- My opinion matters.
- I am a magnet for love.
- Self-love is a natural state of being.
- I am loved, and I am wanted.
- I think positive thoughts about myself and other persons.
- I protect myself against any hurt that comes through my way
- I just like the person I see in the mirror
- I will stop apologizing for being myself.
- Negative self-talk is not welcomed in my life.
- I do not bow to my fears.
- My mind, body, and soul are fit and powerful.
- I am grateful for the things I possess.

6 – Weight Loss Affirmations

Easy accessibility to unhealthy foods has created an epidemic all over the world.

The temptation to choose convenience over health is hard to beat.

Myriads of persons struggle with weight-loss, going back and forth between diets, but never discover success.

If that is you or you are simply looking to enhance your diet and overall health, these affirmations are certainly for you.

- ➢ I love all the things about my body.
- ➢ I am thankful for how effectively and efficiently my body functions.
- ➢ I am very grateful and excited that I weigh much lesser now.
- ➢ I crave healthy, nutritious foods.
- ➢ I so much love the taste of fruits and vegetables.
- ➢ I am in love with each cell in my body.
- ➢ I accept the shape of my body and I find it attractive and appealing.

- I only make healthy and nourishing eating choices.

- I take care of my body and exercise each day.

- My body is healthy and full of strength and energy.

- My body is crammed with healing energy whenever I inhale.

- I radiate confidence and other people respect me.

- Others find me sexy and desirable.

- I am filled with happiness when I look in the mirror.

- I feel safe and comfortable in my body.

- I am becoming fitter and stronger each passing day through exercise.

- I am easily reaching and maintaining my desired weight

- I love and care for my body so much.

- I am filled with love, hope, and confidence.

- I am thankful for the life force and energy that runs through my body.

- Each action I take increases my confidence.

- Everything I think, say and do enable me to be healthier.

- I am worthy of having a slim, healthy, attractive body.

- I choose to exercise.

- I love my body.

- I am patient with creating my better body.

- I am excitedly exercising every morning when I wake up so that I can reach the weight loss that I have been wanting.

- I want to eat foods that enable me to look and feel good.

- I am responsible for my health.

7 – Stress Relief Affirmations

Stress relief affirmations often go a long way to calm yourself down.

After all, we all have our bad days.

That does not make us any less of a functioning adult compared to other persons.

Rather than focusing on the things that are stressing you out; though, train your eyes to stay fixed on your goal.

This way, you can bounce right back no matter the number of setbacks you experience along the way.

The following are a list of stress affirmations that work greatly:

> Being calm and centered is one of the utmost priorities in my life.
> I am practicing this feeling.
> I am breathing slowly and deeply, filling myself with a lot of calmness.
> I am worthy of a peaceful and loving life.
> I give myself a credit whenever I do something that makes me excited.

- ➢ I am relaxing and feeling a lot sleepier.
- ➢ I am comfortable around other persons.
- ➢ I let go of defensiveness and choose to fill my world with joy and kindness rather.
- ➢ I forgive with love and let go of the past.
- ➢ I am thankful for the good in my life.
- ➢ I love myself for who I am.
- ➢ I am relaxed and calm.
- ➢ My tension is melting away.
- ➢ I am letting go of all my worries and fears.
- ➢ My mind is slowing down.
- ➢ I am centered and quiet.
- ➢ My muscles are relaxed.
- ➢ My thoughts are calming down.
- ➢ Calmness washes over me with each deep breath I take.
- ➢ I am releasing every negative emotion from my system.
- ➢ I am releasing my concerns by breathing slowly and deeply.
- ➢ Challenges bring opportunities.

> I view stressful situations as challenges.

> I find love and support internally and externally.

> I am calm and relaxed in every situation.

8 – Anxiety Affirmations

Everyone experiences anxiety from time-to-time.

Anxiety and the fears that lead to them are a natural reaction to a big, bad scary world.

Anxiety is natural; it is among our fight or flight response.

Anxiety is our body's way of telling us that something is going to occur and to get ready to run or club something to death.

Unfortunately, our modern society does not permit us to club our problems to death.

And running from a board meeting that gets you anxious may not be nearly as bad a response.

This entails that positive thinking exercises to get rid of your anxious feelings may be one of the best ways to fight anxiety.

Saying your day to day motivational messages a day will decrease anxiety and brighten your day.

The following are a list of affirmations for anxiety

- ➢ Change gives me an opportunity.
- ➢ I am calm, patient, and in total control of my emotions.

- The more I give, the more I will be able to receive.
- My negative thoughts and self-images are gone.
- My strength is stronger than my anxiety.
- I follow my dreams with a lot of vigor.
- The little things in life make all the distinctions.
- I enjoy being surrounded by other people.
- My fear goes down as I live my life with courage.
- I can go with the flow.
- I am excited, healthy, and centered.
- I move above stress to peace.
- My thoughts are positive and full of joy.
- I breathe, I am collected, and I am calm.
- I am safe, and all things are good in my world.
- Inside me, I feel calm, and nobody can disrupt this peacefulness.
- I am freeing myself from fear, judgment, and doubt;
- I choose only to think nice thoughts;
- I am safe. I trust life, and I trust in myself.
- My life is an adventure.

- I recognize that my negative thoughts are irrational, and I am now going to get rid of these fears.
- This is just one moment in time;
- I am not going to be scared by a feeling.
- My anxiety does not control my life. I do.

9 – Dealing with Fear Affirmations

These positive affirmations are designed to assist you to overcome a fear of failure and transform into a person who just goes after success full out with confidence and enthusiasm.

You can repeat these affirmations whenever you desire a boost of confident energy to just go after something without overthinking or worrying.

The positive statements will combat any negativity or fear and keep your mind focused on taking action.

And not only are they effective in the short term, but they can as well be utilized on a daily basis to gradually reprogram your mind for long term change.

You will become a person that is just naturally fearless in the face of challenge, eagerly goes for success with confidence, and accepts setbacks as natural steps on the road to gain ultimate success.

The following are affirmations for dealing with fear:

> ➢ I trust my inner wisdom and intuition.

> ➢ I inhale calmness and exhale nervousness.

> ➢ This situation works out for my utmost good.

- Wonderful things unfold before me.
- Every experience in my life nurtures and supports me.
- I focus on breathing and grounding myself.
- Following my intuition and my heart keeps me safe and sound.
- I make the right choices all the time.
- I draw from my internal strength and light.
- I trust myself.
- As I challenge my fears, I am strengthened and empowered.
- As I challenge my fears, I release my desire to dwell on them.
- Being fearless is one of the highest priorities in my life, and I practice this feeling each passing day.
- I accept that fear is simply a feeling which will subside as I move further.
- I accept that a lot of my fears only exist in a fictitious future that I have created in my imagination.
- I act in spite of the fear and therefore the fear fades away.

- I permit the courage of my heart to dissolve any fears I experience.
- Each day I bravely expand my comfort zone.
- All the things in my life are safe and secure.
- Facing my fears gives me the power to rise beyond them.
- Fear is nothing quite an emotion I permit myself to feel.
- I accept and love my fear, and then I let it go.
- I am conquering my trepidations each day.
- I am daring in everything I do.
- I am fearless every time.
- I am fearless in everything I do.
- I always act in spite of any fears I may have.
- I usually take positive action in the face of fear.
- I am always eager to try new things.
- I am finally freed from all disempowering fears and doubts.
- I am in total control and do not have anything to fear.
- I am in total control of my thoughts and feelings.
- I am in control of which life experiences I choose.

10 – Self Confidence Affirmations

Of all the various areas of your life where positive affirmations can make a difference, the most important area is in your confidence.

As noted earlier, affirmations work by taking negative thoughts, such as doubts, fears, and anxieties and gradually turning them into more positive emotions.

The following are a list of affirmations that will help you with your self-confidence.

> ➤ I am not afraid to be wrong.
>
> ➤ Happiness is within my grasp.
>
> ➤ I am confident in the presence of other people.
>
> ➤ Success will be my driving force.
>
> ➤ The success of others will certainly not make me jealous. My time is now.
>
> ➤ I will speak with a lot of confidence and self-assurance.
>
> ➤ All things will work out for me.
>
> ➤ I am a winner.
>
> ➤ The tools I require to succeed are in my possession.
>
> ➤ There is nobody better to urge the work done than me.

- Other persons will not take advantage of me.

- I have confidence in my skills.

- I will mention "No" when I do not possess the time or inclination to act.

- The only one that is able to defeat me is myself.

- I dare to be different.

- I have faith in my social skills.

- I continue because I think in my path.

- It is always too early to give up on my goals.

- I must know what awaits me at the top of this rope so I do not hand over.

- I possess the courage to make a positive change in my life.

- I acknowledge my very own self-worth; my self-confidence is rising.

- Others look up to me as a pacesetter due to my confidence

- Each day I will be more confident, powerful, and successful

- Feeling confident, assured, and powerful is a normal part of my everyday life

- I am self-reliant, creative and protracted in whatever thing I do.

- I am valuable and can make powerful contributions to the planet today.

- My every desire is achievable.

- Even outside my comfort zone, I will certainly be comfortable in my very own skin.

- If I fail, I will fail forward.

- My confidence knows no bound.

- I cannot hand over until I have tried every conceivable means.

- Giving up is straightforward and always an option so let's delay it for an additional day.

- I made decisions based on the superstar I am emerging.

11 – Self Esteem Affirmations

Positive self-esteem affirmations are useful to enhance confidence and they also assist counter negative thoughts.

Affirmations can seriously assist you to boost self-esteem and help you feel good about yourself.

We have all in one way or the other heard about positive affirmations for self-esteem.

There are many great self-esteem affirmations you will tell yourself daily to assist you to increase your self-esteem.

The following are self-esteem affirmations

- ➤ I always see the best in other persons.
- ➤ I believe in who I am.
- ➤ I am consistent in the things that I say and do.
- ➤ I appreciate everything I possess. I live in joy.
- ➤ I am courageous.
- ➤ I am ready to act in spite of any fear.
- ➤ I make my choice of friends who approve of me and love me.
- ➤ I surround myself with people that treat me well.

- I take the time to show my friends that I care about them.
- My friends do not judge me, nor do they influence what I do with my life.
- I take great pleasure from my friends, even if we argue or live different lives.
- I release negative feelings and thoughts about myself;
- I am positive and optimistic. I believe things will usually transform for the best.
- It is easy to make friends. I attract positive and kind folks into my life.
- It is easy to meet people. I create positive and supportive relationships.
- I am a powerful creator. I create the life I desire.
- I am comfortable as I am. I accept and love myself.
- I am confident. I trust myself.
- I am successful at this time.
- I treat everyone with a lot of kindness and respect.
- I breathe in confidence and breathe out fear.
- I am flexible. I adapt to change quickly.

- ➢ I have integrity. I am entirely reliable. I do what I say.
- ➢ I am competent, smart and capable.
- ➢ I believe in myself,
- ➢ I recognize the many good qualities I possess.
- ➢ I am a passionate person. I am outrageously enthusiastic and inspire other persons.
- ➢ I am calm and peaceful.
- ➢ I possess unlimited power at my disposal.
- ➢ I am kind and loving. I am compassionate and truly care for others.
- ➢ I am focused and persistent. I will never give up.
- ➢ I am energetic and enthusiastic. Confidence is my second nature.

12 – Happiness Affirmations

Happiness is simply a journey, not a destination and happiness affirmations are your companion during this wonderful journey.

These affirmations will assist you in your search for happiness.

Happiness is determined by our attitude toward life.

Two different persons can have a different feeling in a similar situation, counting on their perspective.

For instance, after completing a particularly difficult task, one person may feel relieved that 'work' has been completed.

Another person may be excited that he has completed his task satisfactorily.

One is relieved, the order is happy, the following are happiness affirmations

> ➢ I live my life with gratitude and happiness.
> ➢ I am thankful for the beautiful things in my life.
> ➢ Happiness is my every moment and everyday choice.
> ➢ I am happy, healthy, and grateful.
> ➢ I choose happiness and joy every moment.

- Each day I attract circumstances and situations that overwhelm me with joy.
- I choose to be happy all the time.
- Happiness is my birthright.
- No matter what occurs today, I will find the positive in it.
- I awaken gratefulness for today and that I choose happiness.
- Even in hard times, I choose to see the good in life.
- When I count every blessing in my life I find that I am naturally happy.
- Happiness is alchemy for my spirit.
- Happiness is a natural response to being thankful.
- My natural state is happiness and joy. I reside there.
- I am happy by choice.
- When you ask me the reason I am happy, I answer...let me count the ways...
- I enjoy a lifetime of happiness, health, and harmony.
- My life is filled with happiness, peace, and love.

- Happiness, health, and harmony are the life on behalf of me.
- Many of life's simple pleasures bring me great excitement.
- I can choose to be happy whenever I desire.
- I will search for ways to bring happiness to other people.
- May all beings all over the world, including me, be happy.
- I choose to be happy even in hard times.
- May my happiness be a gift to my friends and my family.
- I am free to choose to be happy.
- My life of joy starts now.
- A lifetime of happiness is cultivated every moment and every day.
- I am happy and I know so I show it.
- The planet deserves nothing but my authentic happiness.
- Let us live in such a way that our happiness is beneficial to the entire world.

13 – Gratitude Affirmations

Gratitude affirmations will assist you to express gratitude for the very life that you are living. Gratitude is the foremost of all human emotions.

The one emotion that transcends all others is gratitude.

In life, it is impossible to form a reciprocating gesture for everything that we receive – intangible or physical.

Not only it is impossible to pay for everything that we get, but most of the days' mere payment does not fully compensate for what we have received.

When one is in a state of thankfulness (gratitude), the body is full of beneficial chemicals.

Also, according to the law of attraction, one attracts only those things or situations in life that one inherently is.

The following are a list of affirmations for gratitude:

> ➢ I am so grateful to be alive.
> ➢ I am grateful for every day.
> ➢ I am so blessed for everything I possess.
> ➢ Gratitude grounds me to this moment.

- I find gratitude in each experience.

- I find gratitude and joy each day.

- I am grateful for all the blessings I possess.

- I live my life with awareness and gratitude.

- I choose to be thankful regardless of the circumstances.

- I am thankful for the Universe and all of her abundance.

- Life offers me abundant blessings to be grateful for.

- I cannot wait to begin the day.

- I embrace today with open arms

- I am prepared for a new day filled with opportunities

- I align myself with joy, peace, and prosperity

- I am aware of my body's strength and capabilities

- I am capable and calm in any situation

- I am full of vitality and I love my life

- I find something to be grateful for each day.

- Every day blesses me with more things to be grateful for.

- Gratitude in challenging times assists me to grow.

- Thank you for another day.

14 – Forgiveness Affirmations

Forgiveness is simply a virtue of the warrior spirit.

It is like taking a giant weight off your shoulders and the other individual does not necessarily have to change, say "thank you," or otherwise.

It is no one's duty but yours to clear out negative feelings and resentment, and your body-mind will thank you.

Here are some good affirmations to assist wash away the pain of resentment to a more loving, fresher, cleaner and joyful life.

> ➤ I release the pain of anger and rage from my entire body.

> ➤ I release my past and forgive my participation in it.

> ➤ I accept my past and learn from it.

> ➤ I practice understanding and compassion.

> ➤ I am free from every prison of resentment.

> ➤ Resentment replicates old turmoil and I choose my life to be free from drama.

> ➤ I do not confuse people from my past with people within the present.

> ➤ I acknowledge my faults and forgive myself totally.

- I make peace (inside) with anyone who has done me wrong.
- Forgiveness is a gift to myself.
- My parents did the best they could. I sincerely forgive them for any wrong that they unknowingly did and forgive myself for holding a grudge against them.
- When I forgive myself, it becomes easier to forgive other persons.
- Forgiveness offers me a fresh start and a clean slate.
- I forgive to stop the negative karmic cycle in my life.
- Every day is filled with new possibilities.
- The past is gone. I now live in the present.
- I am the architect of my future.
- I am a pioneer of the future and certainly not a prisoner of the past.
- I am forgiving, loving, gentle and kind to everybody.
- I put down the heavyweight of doubt, guilt, embarrassment, and self-hate.
- Intention is my catalyst for my ideal future.

- I am able to move beyond my very own mistakes.

- I am able to heal from the hurt of my past.

- I am worthy of all the compassion and kindness on this planet.

- I will treat myself with so much love and respect.

- I love myself and all that I am.

- I go with the flow.

- I grow more patient and understanding of other persons by forgiving myself.

- I cease all self-judgment and self-sabotage.

- I forgive myself each day at a time.

- I did the best I could at the time with what I knew.

- I have the boldness to heal any wound.

15 – Let Go Affirmations

Learning how to let go is not often easy.

Many folks have trouble saying goodbye to painful memories, a person we have lost or anger we are holding onto.

We may even discover some comfort in the familiarity of rehashing those stories or feelings, even though they weigh us down.

And letting go is not often about the past; we usually struggle to release the future too.

Sometimes I see myself worrying about what is going to occur tomorrow or pondering about what I can do to control the outcome of a certain situation.

I think most of us can relate to that on some level, whether it occurs here and there... or perhaps much more frequently.

Below is a list of letting go affirmations that will assist you:

> ➢ I feel special knowing that I am a part of something bigger, which has meaning above my wildest dreams.

> ➢ Success and luck flow in my direction in a river of abundance.

- Opportunities and advantages accompany each door that I open.
- Every day I feel and hook up with the gorgeous spirit that I am.
- Each day I make a choice to search and acknowledge my personal happiness.
- I am usually all that I need to live a joyful life.
- Tomorrow is a precious gift that I am thankful for.
- I choose how I feel, and I feel amazing.
- My future is better than I could ever think of.
- I am thankful for each day that brings me one step closer to my perfect life.
- I see miracles in each day.
- No one loves me more than myself.
- I am thankful for a new day to play in.
- I see perfection in the natural world all around me.
- I love that I feel so joyful.
- I enjoy sharing my life with supportive friends and family.

- All the things I desire in life are in front of me.

- I rejoice in the process of creating positive change in my life.

- The future is mine. All I need to do is to claim it.

- I open myself up to the happiness that every day can bring.

16 – Be in Place Affirmations

Even if you do not have young children running all over the place, peace and calm are often hard to return by.

There are a lot of disruptive forces in our modern lives, and our busy minds begin to babble as a cause.

There is the nonstop ping of technology, Daily commutes, Stressful workplace and the world at large, egad—terrorism, election, Wall Street, climate change.

The following list of affirmations will assist you to overcome these disruptive forces:

- ➢ There is an honest reason I used to be paired with this perfect family.
- ➢ I choose to view my family as a gift.
- ➢ I am a far better person from the hardship that I have scaled through with my family.
- ➢ I love and accept myself.
- ➢ I release every negative energy that is holding me back.
- ➢ I permit myself to take some time off.
- ➢ I know my wisdom guides me to the proper decision.

- I am trustworthy to make the best decision for myself.
- I receive all feedback with so much kindness but make the ultimate call myself.
- I listen lovingly to the present inner conflict and reflect thereon until I get to peace around it.
- I love my family albeit they do not understand me totally.
- I am comfortable and satisfied with myself.
- I am stress and worry-free.
- I am surrounded by peace and quietness.
- My mind is quiet and stress-free.
- My body feels calm and light.
- I am at peace with myself and therefore the world around me.
- Nothing hinders me from feeling calm and peaceful.
- Life is beautiful and calm.
- My breath is slow and relaxed.
- I show my family the extent I love them all together with the verbal and non-verbal ways I can.
- I feel joy and ease at this particular moment.

17 – Personal Growth Affirmations

Everyone is on an endless path of spiritual growth whether we know it or not.

This includes you.

Some days (weeks, months, and even years) we may feel stunted or at a standstill.

Perhaps feel as if you're spinning your wheels, not moving forward.

Each experience (the good, the bad, and the ugly) gives us the chance to stretch a bit and ultimately soar to recent heights.

It is how you approach the good times and bad times that will give rise to or deflate your momentum.

Utilizing supportive affirmations can assist you to reach up and meet your potential.

They can offer you the boost you need to remain focused on your path and keep your momentum soaring.

> ➤ I am committed to becoming the person I desire to become.

- My mind is like water. I will change and adjust as required.
- I will master distractions and maintain my focus on my goals.
- I am committed to improving my life.
- I will achieve every one of my goals.
- I have an idea of action to achieve my desires.
- My priorities are clear. I work to finish my most vital tasks first.
- My goals are my focus.
- I am becoming the most ideal version of myself.
- I see adversity as opportunities to grow.
- I choose to exchange the word failure with opportunity
- Each day, in every way, I am growing
- I am gentle and forgiving of myself
- I am compassionate, kind, and patient with myself
- It is in the brokenness that I am healing
- I am elevating onward and upward
- I am capable of doing anything I put my mind on

- ➤ I find new opportunities to assist me to grow

- ➤ Nothing will stand in my way.

- ➤ I will overcome any challenges.

- ➤ I anticipate facing challenges as opportunities to grow.

- ➤ I am so resilient and strong

- ➤ I have faced challenges previously and overcome them

18 – Love Affirmations

If you would like to attract love in your life, you got to first give out love.

The affirmations for love provided here will assist you to become a loving person.

Humans cannot survive in the absence of food, air, water, and love.

As you can see, among the four indispensable things of life, love is solely intangible.

Discover love in your life using these positive affirmations for love.

Love takes a lot of forms.

The love between a mother and her baby, the love between two friends, between two lovers, between two life partners and so on.

So we see in our society that when folks are unable to seek love among humans, many tend to adopt pets.

Thus, in a single form or another, love must exist in life.

The ideal way to receive love the way you desire is to shower it an equivalent way on those whom you love.

Love affirmations will assist you in your endeavor.

> ➤ I radiate love and other persons reflect love back to me.
>
> ➤ I am loving and lovable.
>
> ➤ I am attractive.
>
> ➤ My romantic relationship is long-lasting, healthy, and filled with love.
>
> ➤ Every communication between my partner and I is loving and kind.
>
> ➤ Everything about me is lovable and deserves love.
>
> ➤ I am with my soul mate because I am a loving, kind one that deserves true love.
>
> ➤ I awake each morning crammed with joy because I do know that I face every day with the support and love of my partner.
>
> ➤ I am surrounded by love and everything is great.
>
> ➤ My partner finds me sexy because (he/she) is interested in every part of me.
>
> ➤ All of my relationships are been healthy because they are based on love and compassion.

- My partner is so kind, compassionate and understanding.

- My partner is extremely physically and spiritually interested in me.

- I am with my soul mate and we share a life overwhelmed with love.

- Life is filled with love and I discover it everywhere I go.

- My relationship is divine, and my partner and I are a perfect match.

- There is an in-depth understanding between my partner and that me.

- Forgiveness and compassion are the bedrock of my romantic relationship.

- It is easy for me to look through the mirror and say, "I love you."

- My words are always kind and loving, and reciprocally, I hear kindness and love from other persons.

- Every day of my life is overwhelmed with love.

19 – Relationship Affirmations

No matter how intense love begins, after a particular period of time, the "honeymoon" wears off.

Thankfully, that energy can change into other things – appreciation and respect, a deeper love, more understanding, and a little conflict, and more oneness and less separateness.

We are not taught classes on character qualities and ideals, love and relationships, or maybe conscious communication in our college system, so it is no wonder why we fail so miserably at relationships and marriages.

There are, however, numerous great ways we can sustain a loving relationship; one among them being daily affirmations.

Saying these affirmations reminds us to require responsibility for our thoughts, feelings, and actions and sets the correct intention to possess an enduring, harmonious relationship.

- ➢ I act from a place of love.
- ➢ I have a lot of trust for my partner.
- ➢ I know my partner is making good decisions.
- ➢ I believe in my partner.
- ➢ Trust for my partner is growing stronger every day.

- My partner loves and trusts me.

- I respect my partner a lot.

- My partner acts with integrity.

- I communicate in a loving way with my partner.

- I respect and appreciate my partner so deeply.

- I can comfortably express my needs and feelings.

- I am free to be myself in my relationship.

- I am in a secure and loving relationship.

- I am loved, cherished and taken good care of.

- I am perfectly able of understanding my partner`s needs.

- I believe in the strength of my relationship.

- I am entirely aligned with my partner.

- Our relationship is getting stronger every day.

- My love for my partner grows every day.

- Our relationship will last long.

- I respect my partner`s boundaries.

- I am considerate of my partner`s feelings.

- I am in a loving and lasting relationship.

- I will make this relationship work.

- ➤ Our relationship is strong and whole.
- ➤ We will stick together all through our lives.

20 – Friendship Affirmations

Most persons find making new friends difficult especially making friends as an adult.

Friendship is a really vital contributor to mental wellbeing and happiness so it is a necessary thing to find out the way to do.

Affirmations are an excellent way to make sure you have the proper mindset when setting out to achieve any goal also as being a constant reminder of why you started.

The following are a list of friendship affirmations:

- I trust myself, I trust life, and that I trust my friends.
- Loving others is easy once I love and accept myself.
- I have an in-depth connection with my friends.
- I attract friends with ease.
- I make choices of friends who approve of me and love me.
- I surround myself with persons that treat me well.
- I am deserving of love and respect.
- I am worthy of friendship and companionship.
- I enjoy chatting with my work colleagues.
- I like getting to know new individuals.

- Everyone I meet this day is warm and friendly.

- I am adequate as I am to be loved as an honest friend.

- I permit myself and persons around me to be imperfect.

- I love and accept myself, and that I am a magnet for friends.

- I know that the friend I want at each moment in my life will appear with perfect timing.

- I take the time to point out to my friends that I care about them.

- My friends do not judge me, nor do they influence what I do with my life.

- I harmoniously resolve conflicts with my friend for the highest good within every one of us.

- My friends are a means of happiness in my life.

- I like who I am.

- I am surrounded by the love of friends.

- I feel safe and comforted by my friends.

- I permit my friends to be who they are and the way they are within the moment.

➤ I take great pleasure in my friends, albeit we disagree or live different lives.

➤ I have healthy boundaries.

➤ I am able to open my heart to true friendship and a meaningful connection.

➤ I am allowed to mention 'no' to requests for me to do favors for people and still deserve good friendship.

➤ I am grateful for my friends.

➤ I am attracting kind, warm and friendly persons into my life.

➤ I believe in the entire goodness of people.

➤ I am a good friend to my neighbors.

21 – Money Affirmations

Make use of these money affirmations to draw in wealth in your life.

I have been hooked into affirmations and I utilize them each day in my life.

I have a list of various affirmations for money.

The law of attraction states that each positive or negative event that happened with you was attracted by you.

Rehearsing money affirmations each day will assist change your life for the better and manifest wealth towards your life.

Fix in your mind the precise amount of cash you desire and begin thinking positive thoughts in your mind to draw in abundance.

➢ Money flows with ease

➢ I can feel it

➢ Money comes unexpectedly

➢ Money comes in great frequency and huge numbers.

➢ I am worthy and deserving of money

➢ Wealth is my birthright

- Money flows with ease to me
- My financial freedom is just one step away
- It is flowing to me
- There is more than enough to go around
- Everything I desire is coming to me
- I cannot wait to get more
- I am rich
- I am wealthy
- I am financially librated
- I am receiving more and more
- I know I deserve more
- Money is a source of energy, as am I
- Money loves me.
- It is attracted to me
- I am blessed

22 – Abundance /Prosperity Affirmations

We need abundance to free ourselves from material worries, we need them to supply all the great things to our loved ones, and that we need them to pursue our deepest passions.

Unfortunately, many of us have false beliefs that cash is bad, that rich folks are evil, that living the abundant life is not for the regular man or woman, that enormous ambitions are literally bad for the character.

On the opposite side; people who indeed respect money and need to have them in abundance, they simply lack the power to believe themselves.

They think that their education was not adequate, they believe they lack sufficient talent, or there is no adequate time for earning that much money...

All of these and other beliefs possess their deepest roots since our most youthful years and we do not have an idea of where they have come from.

You must understand that everything you think about prosperity and abundance is simply a mirrored image of other people's beliefs, opinions, and attitudes.

The following are a list of affirmations that will help you receive abundantly:

- ➤ My passion is the secret to my abundance.
- ➤ Wealth is pouring into my life.
- ➤ I am getting wealthier every day.
- ➤ I enjoy travel whenever I want.
- ➤ I am successful in anything I do.
- ➤ I am consistently adding to my income.
- ➤ I always have enough money for all the things I desire.
- ➤ I am wealthy above my wildest dreams.
- ➤ I am deserving of abundance
- ➤ I am grateful for all I do possess and so thankful for all that is coming
- ➤ What an amazing life I live
- ➤ I enjoy an abundance of money.
- ➤ I clearly see opportunities to make cash effortlessly.
- ➤ I feel great concerning loving money.
- ➤ Money loves me; I now have more than I desire
- ➤ I am so blessed to possess this level of wealth

- I am so blessed to attain this position
- The universe brings me fulfillment and abundance.
- Everything I touch is a success.
- Money flows to me easily, frequently and abundantly.
- I utilize money to make the planet a far better place.
- I enjoy multiple streams of passive income.

23 – Career Affirmations

Searching for a new job is like searching for a new relationship.

We do not do it frequently and when we do, we are a little out of practice.

Other persons are happy in their current job but want to make it more fulfilling.

These affirmations are written to assist you to build the confidence you can and also the fulfillment you seek in your present job.

- My recent business income will continue to grow.
- I am calm and confident.
- New opportunities come to me with ease.
- I will attract positive customer.
- When opportunity knocks, I will be able to answer the door.
- I deserve my best job and this day I find it
- Each time I interview, I exude energy and confidence
- Each time I interview, I exude capability and credibility
- Whenever I interview, I always impress

- I am ready for my interviews. I am confident in my interviews.
- I am successful in my interviews.
- Good jobs are appearing in my life out of nowhere
- As I put my intention for an excellent job out into the Universe, the Universe responds with excellent job opportunities.
- I am creating my dream career. It appears in my mind then in my world.
- Career change is a chance to have the career I desire. This time I choose an excellent career for me
- No more excuses! I deserve a job that fulfills me and now I am prepared to find it
- Right this moment, my resume is being seen by all the appropriate personalities.
- My resume provides me interviews and I show up to seal the deal
- Right now, the job I am searching for is searching for me

- ➤ I am recession-proof! I possess the skills and therefore the talent to compete in any economy

- ➤ I am a great employee! Any employer is fortunate to have me

- ➤ I am an asset to any organization and I prove it in all interviews.

- ➤ My confidence is building! My ideal career arrives in my life this day

- ➤ My perfect job is on a direct collision course with me this moment

- ➤ I committed to my happiness in this job search and my determination pays off

- ➤ I am ready to work! I am ready to contribute! I communicate that energy in each interview

- ➤ Every no for my wrong job gets me closer to the yes that is right for me

- ➤ I close my eyes and I see myself in my right job. I open my eyes and I go make it happen

- Breathing in, I know I am deserving of an excellent career. Breathing out, I have it

- The negative news about jobs is about averages. I am beyond average

24 – Business Affirmations

A part of you is tired in the restriction and limitations your present "money" situation has you in and you are prepared to make major moves in your business to enable your dreams to come true.

Making money together with your business is not solely knowing what to do.

It really comes down to knowing the appropriate thing to do in the right order and having the mental stamina to see it through.

It requires positivity, consistent action, focus, perseverance, and a moneymaker mindset; because if you do not truly believe you will be able to achieve those big money goals you set annually, no action you ever take will create the long-term success you wish for.

The following are a list of business affirmations:

> I am grateful for the opportunities that come my way

> I am thankful for each and every person who added to the success of my business

> I am smart and successful

> I am able to achieve any goals I set myself in business

- ➢ I create great business opportunities
- ➢ My income is constantly improving
- ➢ My business is an enormous success
- ➢ I believe in myself and trust in my abilities to succeed in everything I do
- ➢ Being successful is natural for me
- ➢ Success, money, and happiness comes to me with ease
- ➢ My work makes a difference
- ➢ My business allows me to possess a life I really like
- ➢ I am energized in my business
- ➢ I love the liberty my business provides for me
- ➢ My business dreams are manifesting incessantly
- ➢ I am a good match for my ideal business
- ➢ My income is increasing rapidly
- ➢ As I become more and more successful, I assist more and more persons
- ➢ I am so passionate about my business and that indicates in everything I do
- ➢ I attract sales with ease

- I attract my ideal clients with ease

25 – Work Affirmations

Work is a common area where myriads of individuals want to improve and get ahead.

People might want to get promotions in their 9-5 jobs.

They may want to look for a job that possesses security.

They may need a new job where they are challenged and can grow with the company.

They may want to turn their side hustle into its personal viable business.

There are a lot of reasons why people want to get ahead in a job, but the reasons do not count.

Positive daily affirmations will assist them to get there.

Obviously, affirmations on their own are not going to enhance your productivity at work.

However, the increased energy and positive mindset from the affirmations will enable a big impact on your personal productivity.

The following are a list of positive work affirmations to use:

- I further my career with each action I take.

- I have my dream job.

- I love each day I work.

- My career brings me closer to my family.

- My job brings me financial abundance.

- My colleagues love being around me.

- I will work smarter, not harder.

- I am a positive influence, and I surround myself with other persons like me.

- Time is my most valuable asset. I protect my time carefully.

- Balance is key. I will mix self-care with effort.

- My progress is always going forward.

- My boss values the work I do.

- I am a valued employee.

- My clients appreciate and value my work.

- I attract new clients each passing day.

- I feel free to give myself the TLC I desire.

- Positive energy surrounds me.

- My positive attitude, confidence, and diligence naturally draw in recent opportunities.
- I am rewarded for doing my very best.
- I engage in healthy stimulation during my break time.
- I eat healthy, nutritious food during my lunch break and my body is excited, granting me energy and healthiness reciprocally.
- I radiate success.
- I am enthusiastic and happy about my work.
- My career is one of my dreams.
- When I say "no" to the incorrect job, I move that much closer to the right career.
- My enthusiasm concerning my job is contagious.
- My workplace is peaceful and filled with so much love.
- I make decisions with ease
- I speak positively about my colleagues and they respond by speaking positively concerning me.
- I am a wonderful employee. Any company would be fortunate to have me.

26 – Success Affirmations

A lot of persons often refer to success with the idea that success = money.

It can be that, but there are a lot of ways to be successful.

If relationships are your goal, having a happy, healthy family is a success.

If traveling is your goal, visiting a lot of places and checking off hundreds of items from a vibrant bucket list may be the meaning of success.

Only you know what it entails for you to achieve success.

A lot of people are unhappy because they measure themselves utilizing other person's yardsticks for success and perhaps find themselves wanting.

But no matter what you think of as the measure of success, you can tailor your personal affirmations to assist you to achieve that.

The following are success affirmations:

- ➤ Being successful comes to me with ease.
- ➤ I am worthy of financial stability.

- I am open-minded and ready to explore any path leading to success.
- Limiting beliefs have no place in my life. I am optimistic and open-minded.
- Organization comes to me naturally.
- The money I spent comes back to me multiplied.
- I possess all the power I need to make the success I want.
- The universe offers bountiful opportunities for my success.
- I refuse to be distracted from my goals and vision.
- Each day is filled with new ideas and new possibilities.
- I am entirely committed to achieving success in my life.
- My only limit is myself.
- I work well being under pressure and always feel motivated.
- I am living to my full potential.
- I possess everything I want to face any obstacles that surface.
- I control my day; I will not allow my day to control me.

- My passion for business brings tangible results.

- I will not allow others to impose their limitations on me.

- I have the power to make all the success and prosperity I want.

- The universe is crammed with endless opportunities for my career.

- I am surrounded by supportive, positive persons that believe me and need to view my succeed

27 – Religion Affirmations

Religious affirmations are what we use to maintain our faith in God.

They provide us with the feeling that God is always with us and he is fighting all our battles spiritually.

Say them with a lot of faith and see things turn around for good for you in your daily life.

The following is a list of Biblical affirmations:

> The Lord is my light. As dark as this world may appear, I do not have to walk in darkness. Psalm 27:1

> The Lord is present with me, an ever-present help in time of need. Psalm 46:1

> The Lord is coming. He will save me so I don't have to be anxious or afraid. Isaiah 35:4

> I can do everything through Christ who strengthens me. Philippians 4:13

> I am equipped for each good deed and lavished with every grace. II Corinthians 9:8

➤ The Lord is my Shepherd. I lack no good thing. Psalm 23:1

➤ The Lord is my rock and refuge. He will be a safe place for me today. Psalm 18:1

➤ God has filled my life with good things. I can trust Him to satisfy me. Psalm 103:1-5

➤ I am not destined for stumbling or destruction. I have a noble purpose and hope. I Peter 2:8-9

➤ I am precious to God and He will take care of me. Matthew 6:25-44

28 – Spirituality Affirmations

Spiritual affirmations are meant to draw you closer to God.

Read those given below or make your own on similar lines and repeat them alongside prayers.

They can as well be referred to as Affirmations of faith or religion.

Closeness to God is been achieved in a lot of ways.

Praying is one of them and affirmations can be another.

If you are a spiritual person, then you ought to be saying your prayers incessantly.

Prayers ought to be a link between God and therefore the person saying them.

In a similar way, you can repeat one or two (or even more) affirmations along with your prayers.

These affirmations will fine-tune your subconscious mind together with your spirituality.

The advantages are explicit.

The distinction between spiritual and other affirmations is that the previous are non-materialistic.

They are majorly for the enlightenment of the soul.

The following are spiritual affirmations you ought to practice:

- ➢ I am strong enough to overcome negativity.
- ➢ I am more creative to express myself.
- ➢ Every problem is the illusion of the mind.
- ➢ I have the power to accomplish any task I set my mind to with ease and comfort.
- ➢ I give out love and joy, complete presence and openness, toward every being.
- ➢ I focus not on the numerous things I may need to do at some future time, but on the single thing, I can do now.
- ➢ I do not pollute my beautiful, radiant inner being or the world with negativity. I do not offer unhappiness in any form whatsoever a dwelling place inside of me.
- ➢ I perceive other person's body and mind as just a screen, behind which I can feel their true reality; even as I feel mine.

- I am content with what I possess. I rejoice in the way things are. I find out that there is nothing lacking. The entire world belongs to me.

- My peace is so wide and so deep, that anything that is not peace, disappears into it as if it had never been in existence.

- I possess infinite patience when it involves fulfilling my destiny.

- I am a Divine creation, a piece of God. So, I cannot be unworthy.

- I am connected to a vast source of abundance.

- I have access to vast assistance. My strength emanates from my connection to my Source of being.

- I am an infinite being. The age of my body has nothing pertaining to what I do or who I am.

- I relax and do away with all mental burdens, letting God to precise through me His perfect love, peace, and wisdom.

- The healing power of my Spirit is moving around all the cells of my body. I am made of the one universal God-substance.

- God's excellent health flows through the dark nooks of my bodily sickness. In every one of my cells, His healing light is shining. They are totally well, for His perfection is in them.

- Daily I will be capable to search for happiness more and more within my mind, and fewer and fewer through material pleasures.

- God is the shepherd of my restless thoughts. He will direct them to His abode of peace.

- I will make my mind pure with the thought that God is guiding my entire activity.

- Using the sword of devotion, I sever the heart-strings that tie me to delusion. With an in-depth love, I lay my heart at the feet of Omnipresence.

- I reside in this moment by being thankful for all of my life experiences as a toddler.

➢ As I remove complexities in my life, I free myself to answer the callings of my soul.

➢ Being myself has to be with no risks. It is my ultimate truth, and I live fearlessly.

➢ I am submerged in eternal light. It permeates each particle of my being. I am living in that light. The Divine Spirit fills me within and without.

➢ God is within and around me, protecting me; so I will send away the fear that shuts out His guiding light.

➢ I will assist weeping ones to smile by smiling myself, even when it is hard.

29 – Creativity Affirmations

Just imagine that your creativity was just always flowing effortlessly and naturally, and you never felt stumped or at a loss for brand new ideas.

It is very possible to get into a highly creative state, you only need to learn to shift the way you think and adopt the proper mindset for really tapping into your creative energy.

Some of the most vital reasons that creativity does not flow is because we attempt too hard, do not believe ourselves, or cannot just allow our imagination to take over and do its work.

These positive affirmations will assist you with all of this.

With consistent usage, they are going to release your mind and instill positive thought patterns that are conducive to creativity and imagination.

> ➤ I am a creative genius.
> ➤ I am a fount of ingenuity.
> ➤ I am a magnet for new and creative ideas.
> ➤ I am a naturally artistic individual.
> ➤ I am a strong and resourceful creator.

- I am a visionary.
- I permit my creative energy to flow freely every time.
- I always follow the way inspiration leads.
- I frequently have lots of unique ideas for solving problems.
- I am a brilliant and successful artist.
- I am a very creative problem solver.
- I choose to create.
- The artist is already present within me.
- I attract brilliant ideas.
- This day I am making time to create.
- Divine inspiration surrounds me.
- I am awake and see the planet through fresh eyes.
- Being creative enables me to feel so alive.
- I am frequently developing as an artist.
- This day, I am filled with infinite, creative energy.
- My creative being wants to go out and play.
- I am spontaneous; I surprise even myself.
- The wellspring of creativity runs deep.

- An endless reservoir of creativity lies within me.

- My creative strength is limitless.

- I offer myself room for expression.

- Being creative is amongst my utmost joys in life.

- Being creative is one of the highest priorities in my life, and I practice this feeling each day.

- My creativity flows freely.

- I am prepared to share my authentic expression.

- I open myself to a life of creativity.

30 – Fun Affirmations

Feeling down?

I think it is vital to offer ourselves permission to not always be excited, but there are also simple ways to enhance our mood when we are feeling down.

These funny daily affirmations will offer you that much-needed boost to look at things from a fresh perspective and alter your thoughts.

I have had great success utilizing daily affirmations for my personal development.

Make use of these funny affirmations to assist when feeling down.

> Was it a bad day? Or was it a nasty five minutes that you milked all day?

> Some visualize a weed, I visualize a wish

> Compliment people: magnify their strengths, not their weaknesses

> You cannot make everyone excited. You are not a jar of Nutella

> Life is better when you always laugh

- Good things occur once you distance yourself from negativity
- Tell the negative committee that meets inside your head to take a seat down and keep quiet
- Good things will happen this day if you choose to not be a miserable cow
- Giving up on your goal as a result of one setback is like slashing your other three tires because you bought a flat
- Wear your positive pants
- Toss your hair in a bun, placed on some gangster rap, drink some coffee and handle it
- Why choose to be moody when you can shake your booty
- When something does not go appropriately in your life, just yell "plot twist" and advance
- Be a pineapple: stand tall, put on a crown, and be sweet on the inside
- Chin up princess else the crown slips
- If life offers you melons you would possibly be dyslexic
- Not everybody has to like you. Not everyone has taste.

- We are too worried concerning being "pretty" let us be pretty kind, pretty smart, pretty funny, pretty strong.
- Be brace. Even if you are not, pretend to be.
- Get your happy on
- When shit occurs turn it into fertilizer
- I love it when the coffee kicks in and I realize what an adorable badass I am going to be today
- Excuse, I have to go be awesome
- Think like a proton; always positive.
- Tact is the capability to inform a person to travel to hell in such a way that they look forward to the trip
- I am grateful for all those hard persons in my life. They have shown me exactly who I do not want to be
- It is ever too late to urge your shit together
- Be excited; it drives people crazy
- Do not border about those that talk behind your back, they are behind you for a purpose
- Each time you are prepared to find some humor during a difficult situation, you win

Chapter 8: Affirmations for Everyday Life

Morning Affirmations

➢ I am excited to wake up each morning and experience this beautiful life, that I am creating with my thoughts and visions.

➢ Every day is a new beginning. I take a deep breath, I smile, and I start again.

➢ I know each day is a blessing and a gift.

➢ I wake up every morning ready for a new day of exciting possibilities.

➢ I greet this day with confidence and ease.

➢ Today I abandon my old habits and take up new, more positive ones.

➢ I am determined and will never give up.

➢ My life is a blast of growing opportunity because I never stop creating.

- Just one small positive thought in the morning can change my whole day.
- To be positive is to be productive.
- No negative thought will take root in my mind.
- My thoughts do not control me, I control my thoughts.
- My life is a gift. I will use this gift with confidence, joy, and exuberance.
- I am thankful for what I have, even if it is not perfect.
- I am grateful that my life is so happy and successful.
- I believe in my ultimate potential.
- I am fulfilling my purpose in this world.
- I give myself permission to go after what I want.
- My mind and my heart will remain open today.
- Today I align myself with freedom, growth, and joy.
- Today is going to be a really, really good day.
- I release all resistance of the past and move into the present moment.
- Today I focus on what makes me feel good.
- Today I will make progress towards my goals.

- I have everything I need to face any obstacles that come.
- I have the power to create all the success and prosperity I desire.
- I am feeling healthy and strong today.
- Today I love my body fully, deeply and joyfully.
- My body has its own wisdom and I trust that wisdom completely.
- My body is simply a projection of my beliefs about myself.
- I am growing more beautiful and luminous day by day.
- My energy and vitality are increasing every day.
- I open to the natural flow of wellness now.
- Abundant health and wellness are my birthrights.
- Thank you for my strength, my health, and my vitality.
- I love taking good care of myself.
- I am filled with light, love, and peace.
- I treat myself with kindness and respect.
- I don't have to be perfect; I just have to be me.

- Today I give myself permission to be greater than my fears.
- I love myself no matter what.
- I'm proud of all I have accomplished.
- I know that I can master anything if I do it enough times.
- Fear is only a feeling; it cannot hold me back.
- I'm proud of myself for even daring to try; many people won't even do that!
- With a solid plan and a belief in myself, there's nothing I can't do.
- I open to the flow of great abundance in all areas of my life.
- My grateful heart is a magnet that attracts more of everything I desire.
- Prosperity surrounds me, prosperity fills me, prosperity flows to me and through me.
- Today I embrace simplicity, peace, and solace.
- A peaceful heart makes for a peaceful life.

- Peace comes when I let go of trying to control every tiny detail.
- Where peace dwells, fear cannot.
- Today my mission is to be happy and calm.
- Today I open my mind to the endless opportunities surrounding me.
- Opportunities are everywhere if I choose to see them.
- I boldly act on great opportunities when I see them.
- My intuition leads me to the most lucrative opportunities.
- Today I release fear and open my heart to true love.
- I am grateful for the people in my life.
- Thank you for the qualities, traits, and talents that make me so unique.
- I am joyful every day and create joy for others.

Good Luck Affirmations

- All my prospects bring me abundant good fortune.

- Amazing coincidences come into my life on a regular basis.

- At every turn, an opportunity appears before me.

- Endless opportunities appear in my life.

- Every day brings me endless good fortune.

- Every day I am surrounded by an abundance of opportunities.

- Every day I attract lucky happenstances into my life.

- Every day I celebrate my continued good fortune.

- Every day in every way I am attracting more and more good luck into my life.

- Everything I do brings me great success.

- Everything I touch brings me further good fortune.

- Everything is going my way.

- Fantastic new opportunities come into my life every day.

- Fantastic opportunities greet me at every turn.

- Good fortune is one of the top priorities in my life, and I practice this feeling every day.
- Good luck comes to me effortlessly.
- Good luck flows into my life every day.
- Good news visits me regularly.
- Good things keep on happening to me.
- Great things keep blessing my life.
- I affirm abundant good luck throughout my day.
- I always get what I wish for.
- I always land on my feet.
- I always seem to be in the right place at the right time.
- I am a luck magnet.
- I am a magnet for good luck.
- I am a powerful luck magnet.
- I am a vacuum for lucky happenstances.
- I am always 'up' on my luck.
- I am always in the right place at the right time with the right frame of mind.
- I am always prepared. That is why I am so lucky.

- I am constantly drawing good luck with me.

- I am good fortune made flesh.

- I am good luck personified.

- I am incredibly lucky.

- I am lucky in everything I do.

- I am my own good luck charm.

- I am the luckiest man/woman in the world.

- I am the luckiest person alive!

- I am the world's greatest good luck charm.

- I attract good luck into my life by imagining the very best at all times.

- I continuously embed powerful good luck messages into my mind.

- I create my own luck as I go along.

- I create my own luck every day.

- I draw lucky opportunities to me.

- I expect good fortune every moment of my life.

- I expect good luck at all times.

- I expect great things to happen every day of my life.

- I expect the best and I always get it.

- I expect to be lucky every day.

- I feel like the luckiest person alive.

- I feel really lucky today.

- I feel the powerful presence of good luck every day.

- I focus all my attention on the good fortune I desire.

- I focus all my thoughts on good luck, and good luck comes into my life.

- I focus on being lucky at every opportunity.

- I have a good luck charm that never fails me.

- Lady luck is on my side.

- Lady luck loves me today!

- Miracles bless my life every day.

- My good fortune increases every day.

- My good luck charm works for me because I believe in it.

- My good luck is solely a product of my positive thoughts and actions.

- My life is constantly attracting good fortune.

- My positive mindset ensures that I am always lucky.

- I have abundant good luck in all my endeavors.
- I have created a lucky mindset.
- I have empowered my being with infinite good fortune.
- I have the perfect good luck charm; it's called Belief.
- I have trained my mind to create good luck every day.
- I live a charmed life.
- I make my own luck by thinking good fortune at all times.
- I make my own luck by expecting it every day.
- I naturally attract good fortune into my life.
- I practice the feeling of good fortune at every opportunity.
- I see endless opportunities before me.
- I spread good fortune wherever I go.
- I totally believe in luck... that is why it works for me.
- I was born under a lucky star.
- I welcome endless good fortune into my life.
- I welcome serendipity in my life.
- Windfalls come my way regularly.
- With every breath I take, I am bringing more and more luck into my life.

- It's okay for me to have everything I want!

- Every day I grow more financially prosperous

- I always have enough to pay bills and have money leftover

- Abundance flows to me easily and effortlessly

- I'm lucky in life!

- It is my greatest desire to live each and every day with unlimited good fortune.

- Lady luck follows me wherever I go.

- Lady luck is my constant companion.

- My run of good luck is endless.

- My whole life is one lucky streak.

- My world is filled with abundant good luck.

- Serendipity is my constant companion.

- Today I bless my being with limitless good fortune.

- Today I welcome abundant good luck into my life.

- Whomever I meet, good fortune is bestowed upon them.

- My business attracts satisfied customers who keep returning

- From this moment on — I enjoy everything I do

- I am well respected

- My potential is unlimited ... and it shows

- I am the go-to person to get things done, right

- I am even-tempered and well balanced

- Terrific opportunities come to me every day.

- The more I accept good luck, the more of it I experience.

- The smarter I work, the luckier I am.

- Things are going my way!

- Things have a marvelous way of always working out for me.

- Things have an amazing way of always working in my favor.

Empowering Beliefs About Money

Remember: All Prosperity Begins With a Belief in Mind

- ➤ I am good with money when I give it my full attention.
- ➤ I am confident I will learn the skills. I need and find the right people to support me at the right times.
- ➤ I'm confident that I'll be able to afford the help I need at the right times.
- ➤ I am willing to learn and practice new skills, and confident that I will find the support I need at the right times.
- ➤ I am confident in my ability to lead myself toward a successful future, even when that means stepping out of my comfort zone.
- ➤ I can learn everything I need to start, run and grow a successful business.
- ➤ I can learn to network and meet new people in ways that feel rewarding and worthwhile.

- I am great with people.
- I know lots of the right people, and I can meet even more.
- I can relax and enjoy learning new things because it's a necessary part of achieving my dreams.
- I can be successful without becoming a "techie."
- I'll never be too old to try something new and/or be successful.
- I've learned a lot over the years, and I can use all of that to be more successful than.
- I'll never to be too old to pursue my passions and achieve success through them.
- I have many great skills and lots of important knowledge.
- I can make money, and achieve financial success, despite my past experiences.
- I'm confident I can find ways to turn my passions into new ways of making money.
- I deserve lasting financial success and personal fulfillment.
- I like many different people, regardless of their finances.

- I am confident in my ability to make, handle and manage even very large sums of money.
- I want and need a lot of money so that I can enjoy an abundant life, and that includes helping a lot more people.
- I choose to feel relaxed and at ease when I deal with and discuss money.
- I can take calculated risks and achieve financial success without jeopardizing the important things in my life.
- I can take strategic risks and still be a good parent.
- I can start something new and still be available to my kids.
- I am confident that I can pay the mortgage (and more!) doing something I love.
- I'm confident I can manage my health while pursuing something new.
- I'm confident I can find time to try something new.
- I can always make time to finish things.

- I no longer need to limit how much money I'd like to have. I can expand and grow along with my bank balances.
- I deserve and enjoy being noticed for who I am and what I accomplish.
- I already have a pretty good life, and I look forward to welcoming even more abundance into my life.
- I deserve to have good fortune, and there is enough for everyone.
- I can make as much money as I intend to.
- I'm confident that I can manage all the money I make and have complete control over how money flows in and out of my life.
- I can always afford what I want.
- I always make enough money to pay my bills--and a lot more!
- I don't need money to make money.
- Anyone can become skilled at business, including me.

- Perspiration feels great when it comes from doing something I love.
- Success and wealth can and do co-exist with a rewarding and fulfilling personal life.
- Work feels rewarding when I'm doing something I love to do.
- Money is best earned by doing work I love to do.
- Selling is about helping people, and I can learn how to do that in ways that increase sales.
- Even though I don't yet have all the answers, I am confident in my ability to learn any new skills and knowledge I need to succeed.
- Leaders learn about leadership and then test-run what they learn. I can do that, too!
- Lasting financial success is about bouncing back when things don't go as planned. That's part of what I'm learning now.
- Using better tools and systems, I can figure out how to make more money without working too many hours.

- Financial success and personal fulfillment are important to me, so they're worth making time and space in my life.
- When I do work that I love, it's worth it.
- Work that I love fulfills and energizes me.
- Work is rewarding when I'm doing things I love to do.
- It's safe for me to relax and enjoy working with other people.
- People like and respect me for who I am.
- Working with people can be fun, and doesn't have to involve conflict.
- My life is already pretty good, and I'm looking forward to growing and expanding the good in my life.
- Making money is about creating financial abundance, and living up to my potential. It doesn't mean I'm greedy.
- My financial success contributes to others' financial success. This is not a zero-sum game.
- It's safe for me to relax and enjoy interacting with people, both professionally and personally.

➢ Starting something new is exciting! This is important to me, so it's worth the time and effort it requires.

➢ Making money from my passion will make me love it even more.

➢ Hobbies can turn into profitable businesses.

➢ Doing work I love will only make me more productive and successful.

➢ It feels amazing making money doing what I love.

➢ My past experience with money will only help me become wealthier.

➢ Money is a source of joy for me.

➢ Money is pure and abundant.

➢ Rich people are often generous.

➢ Having a lot of money does not affect the kind of person you are.

➢ Rich people are often sincere.

➢ Being successful/having money makes people better versions of themselves.

➢ Anyone, including me, can get rich and famous.

- Having money means being an even better version of myself.
- Making a lot of money means you're helping lots of people.
- When it comes to the rich and middle class, we're all in it together.
- Having money means being able to act on your integrity more often.
- My ever-growing circle of friends and family will still love and appreciate me once I become rich and successful.
- When I make more money, I'll have that much more to gain.
- No amount of money is too much for me. I am confident that I can make and manage financial abundance at a level beyond even my wildest dreams.
- When I think about success, it feels like it is meant to be.
- My kids want me to be happy, which sometimes means investing in myself and my dreams.
- It's not irresponsible to take calculated risks.

- Taking strategic risks in order to pursue my dreams is wise and courageous, not selfish.
- It's perfectly okay for me to want more money.
- Even if it feels scary at first, I'm confident that I can move beyond the fear to pursue my dreams and try new things.
- Making big changes in my life is something I can learn to be comfortable with.
- My life isn't working, which means it's time to go for what I really want.
- In order to fix my life, I need and want to try something new.
- Achieving financial success and personal fulfillment is important to me, so it's worth making time for.
- It's safe for me to achieve success and be noticed for it. I can relax and enjoy an abundant life even more than I enjoy pajamas.
- When I get what I want, I know I can maintain and build on my success.

- Making money is never "a me or them proposition". There's always enough money for everyone.
- My past with money has no effect on how much money I can make now or in the future.
- My gender, race, religion, and cultural heritage do not limit my future success and wealth in any way.
- There is no limit to how much money I can make.
- Being rich is a personal experience, and I can use and spend money however I choose.
- My past education has no bearing on how rich/successful I can become

Leadership Affirmations

- My past education has no bearing on how rich/successful I can become

- I am a thoughtful person and strive to inspire others with my words.

- I am always generous with praise and compliments.

- I inspire others to greatness.

- I inspire others to reach their goals.

- I am an inspiration to others.

- I am an inspiring mentor to others.

- I bring out the best in people.

- I have a magnetic personality.

- I help others to focus on the most positive aspects of themselves.

- I help people to be the best that they can be.

- I inspire and empower others to greatness with my infinite enthusiasm.

- I always encourage others towards their dream.

- I am a born leader.

- I lead others by setting a positive example.
- I am a great visionary.
- I know that I can only lead others where I have been before.
- I set a positive example for others.
- I set trends that others follow.
- I lead others by bringing out the best in them.
- I love being an inspiration to others.
- I remember to thank people often.
- I see the world not as it is, but as it can be.
- My passion for life inspires others.
- With every breath I take, I am bringing more and more charisma into my life.
- With every breath I take, I am bringing more and more magnetism into my life.
- My story of personal freedom inspires others to seek the same.
- My words inspire people all over the world.
- Today I successfully take center stage.

- People trust my opinions and expertise.
- I communicate clearly what I expect of others.
- I take charge easily no matter what the situation.
- People often look to me for advice.
- Making important decisions is just what I do.
- I quickly engage others in teamwork in order to optimize results.
- People recognize me as a leader.
- I am often called on to take charge of a situation.
- I embrace responsibility.
- I eagerly accept new challenges.
- My interpersonal skills are strong.
- I am a good decision-maker.
- People look to me for guidance.
- I am able to take the lead.
- I am a proven leader.
- People always choose me as their team leader.
- Leadership comes naturally to me.
- I have superior leadership skills.

- I make things happen.
- I can draw out the best in others

Bedtime Affirmations for a Beautiful Sleep

- ➤ I can draw out the best in others.

- ➤ I did the best I could today and tomorrow is another day.

- ➤ Thank you for all the blessings of today.

- ➤ Everything that happened today was for my higher good.

- ➤ I am thankful for the people I encountered today.

- ➤ Today, I became a little bit wiser. Thank you.

- ➤ I welcome and embrace the lessons I learned today.

- ➤ I'm proud of myself.

- ➤ I take this moment to see the goodness around me.

- ➤ I let go of any worries or concerns.

- ➤ I take what works from today and leave the rest behind.

- ➤ I am at peace. I am loved.

- ➤ This evening, I feel gratitude and joy.

- ➤ I'm winding down for today and all is well.

- ➤ Tonight I will sleep well and wake up refreshed tomorrow.

- May my sleep be peaceful, may my dreams be filled with love, may my soul awake to the infinite possibilities for happiness in my life.
- I breathe and I will try again tomorrow.
- I'm so thankful for everything I have. Thank you
- I am worthy of love and abundance
- I am confident in myself and know I can accomplish anything.
- I have everything I need to be happy.
- I am thankful for my family and friends.
- I don't need to compare myself to others, I am on my own journey.
- I see the beauty in everyone and everything around me.
- Everything in my life serves my highest good at this time
- I am a healthy, vibrant being of light.
- I release everything that no longer serves me.
- I am the master of my reality.
- I am enough.
- I believe in myself.

- ➢ I love myself.

- ➢ I am at peace.

- ➢ I am now ready to sleep.

Chapter 9

Affirmations for kids

Positive thinking is simply a powerful tool that can enhance your health, assist you to manage stress, overcome challenges, and make good choices.

Everybody can benefit from improving their positive thinking skills.

The idea is that by varying your thinking, you will control your emotions and your actions.

Positive thinking skills often begin with positive-self talk, which entails using the voice in your head to mention positive thoughts concerning yourself or a situation.

Kids could make use of more positive thinking in their lives.

By beginning to think more positively, kids can learn about self believe and work towards their individual potentials.

Kids can utilize a positive affirmation list by reading the words to themselves aloud, discussing how they can assist, and identifying which phrases would work perfectly.

Psychologically, affirmations are rewarding and of great benefit due to the fact that they train us to linger on thoughts we value and defend ourselves with reassurance during threatening situations.

Consistent affirmation practice brings future benefits of self-regulation and emotional management.

We praise our kids frequently for job well done.

But it does not matter if I tell my kids so many times each day how smart, kind, beautiful, and artistic they seem; it is not my opinion and approval that will keep them going in life.

It will be their own belief they possess for themselves, their gifts, and their roles.

It takes some practice but soon weaving brief affirmations into the day to day incessant chatter with kids becomes habit.

We like to add affirmations in our morning ritual and sprinkle them throughout the day during situations that inspire us or that need confidence.

Brain scientists emphasize the importance of specific, repeated positive affirmations done at routine times on a daily basis for at least 21 days.

After that length of your time, the neural connections are being made to coach the brain to think more optimistically.

What to Know when developing a positive self-affirmation habit for kids

It is no secret that a lot of our belief system is made early in life.

Wounds inflicted in childhood can possess far-reaching consequences.

The things we hear from family, friends, and teachers are carried with us throughout our entire lives.

If you seek to develop the positive-affirmation habit in your kids, there are few pertinent things you should have in mind.

1. **Know who your kid is.** Developing positive affirmations ought to be a personal affair. Affirmations should be developed based on your intimate knowledge of each of your children.

2. **You possess a better chance of success when your affirmations are specific and well explanatory.** The way you phrase affirmations plays a role in ensuring their success or failure. You need to make them work. Instead of kids saying "I have many friends", a far better

affirmation would be "I have many friends because I always attempt to assist my friends out once I can."

3. **Positive affirmations can work only if the affirmations are simply realistic.** Avoid unreasonable positive statements. Positive affirmations cannot work if the deeply held negative beliefs are not aligned with the declared affirmations. If the space between the conscious and therefore the unconscious is just too wide, your kids will not end up doing well.

4. **Accept that you might not gain success.** Self-affirmation does not work for everyone. If you discover you are getting negative results, let it go and seek what works well for you.

5. **It takes time to manifest.** The results of self-affirmation are long in coming due to the fact that they require the affirmations to be repeated over an extended period of your time.

6. **Self-affirmation exercises can be an alternative option.** Some studies have indicated that exercises like

writing about what you value can bolster feelings of self-worth. This is less hooked into an individual's self-esteem and is consistent with the thought that grateful kids are more optimistic, happier and more satisfied with their lives.

Precise Steps for Developing a Positive Self-Affirmation Habit in Children

If you would wish to practice self-affirmation together with your kids in the week, here are a couple of simple steps you can attempt:

> ➤ Choose a particular time when you want to practice utilizing self-affirmation and keep it short. Do not make the period too lengthy. Ten minutes a day is quite adequate.

> ➤ Gratitude exercises are simple way to begin. Asking your child to state the items that he/she are grateful for and participating in these exercises is a way to begin. You can set a specified time (for instance a day prior to breakfast or dinner). You can as well offer your child a gratitude journal and keep one yourself.

> ➤ If you prefer to utilize positive affirmations, do not jettison to make them realistic, specific and explanatory. If the affirmations are inconsistent together with your

kids' internal beliefs, they are going to do more harm than good.

➤ Be a model. Children follow the footsteps of their parents. If you would like your kids to begin practicing self-affirmation, they have to observe you practicing it.

➤ Give an explanation to your children why it is vital to develop a positive self-affirmation habit.

➤ Work on a single affirmation at a time. Affirmations only work when they are repeated frequently.

➤ Practice for at least a whole week.

How to Teach Positive Affirmations to Your Kids

The following are ways you can instill positive affirmations in your kids:

Teach Children How to Notice

In making use of positive affirmations for youngsters, it is pertinent to encourage them to first notice if there are any repetitive thoughts already happening.

Explain to your children that repetitive thoughts are like playing a song over and over in their heads. Ask your kids how they listen to music.

What happens once they want to change the song they are listening to?

Do they skip to a subsequent song, download a replacement song or change the radio station?

Discuss how your inner voice works.

We all possess negative thoughts or "songs" we hear inside our heads most times.

Maybe we expect we are not adequate at something or we feel sad.

Other times we have positive thoughts or "songs" we hear with our inner voice that assist us to achieve our goals or feel happy.

If they are playing scary, negative "songs" like: I cannot do this. I am scared. I am not adequate.

I am not beautiful.

I am stupid.

Then, of course, they are going to feel self-doubt, anxiety or anger.

And, if that is the way they are seeing themselves, of course, they will have a hard time seeing the good in the individuals and events around them.

Acknowledge if this is going on and let your kids know that it is normal and that everyone combats those voices.

Encourage your kids to change the negative songs

Explain to your kids that you can change your inner voice and that you are going to imagine changing your inner voice.

Just as we change the song we are listening to, we can as well change our negative thoughts to positive ones.

Positive self-talk can assist us to obtain a positive mindset.

Ask the kids to consider a negative thought or "song" that they have in the mind or had within the mind at just one occasion.

Invite them to change the music.

Lead everyone in miming to show the youngsters the way to change the "songs".

Teach your kids about visualization

It is empowering for kids to act out physically what they are choosing to attempt mentally.

This allows them to disengage with negative thinking and attune instead to a positive affirmation.

Practice not only saying the positive affirmation but as well visualizing themselves completing the goal they need set in a positive, successful way.

As they have the affirmation repeated to themselves, teach them to see themselves that way; reading well, climbing to the top of the jungle gym, making friends, etc.

Offer them some time to notice how imagining it permits them to also feel it in their whole being.

List of Affirmations for Kids

As adults, many of our limiting thought patterns are often attributed to childhood conditioning or having unconsciously adopted negative societal beliefs.

While we search for tactics to assist realign ourselves, how about starting with a far better way forward in our kids?

Most certainly, we can assist our kids with instilling good values, confidence, focus, and belief.

Positive affirmations for kids can do so much to help them in developing healthy self-worth.

We can as well target some for the need of getting an easier time with their school work.

The following is a list of affirmations to make your kids grow with a more positive mindset:

- ➢ I am worthy.
- ➢ I deeply love and accept myself.
- ➢ I enjoy learning.
- ➢ I am divinely protected.
- ➢ I am worthy of affection, trust and kindness.

- I achieve excellent and successful results.

- I am strong.

- I attract like-minded friends easily and naturally.

- I am healthy and am growing up well.

- I am so creative.

- Ideas for solving problems come easily and promptly to me.

- I am a great listener.

- My family, friends and teachers love me for the person I am.

- I am unique and special.

- Each day and in every way, I get better and better.

- My intuition leads me in what I do.

- I experience beauty wherever I go.

- Learning is fun and enjoyable.

- I understand the teachings taught in class totally and on time.

- I believe in myself and my capabilities.

- I learn from my challenges and can often find ways to beat them.
- I am open to possibility.
- I embrace my fears fully and calmly.
- I am calm, relaxed and peaceful.
- I am always within the right place at the proper time.
- I enjoy being, feeling and thinking positive.
- I am loving kindness to everyone.
- I do my best in carrying out my work and tasks.
- I am present.
- I am vibrant and have much energy.
- I possess an awesome imagination.
- I am thankful for my blessings.

Conclusion

Positive Affirmations can be powerful if you know the reason they work so well and how you ought to use them to your advantage.

If you only use positive affirmations as a standalone tool; then chances are that they will not work for you.

The fact is that positive affirmations only scratch the surface of your subconscious mind.

So, if you only make use of positive affirmations, this entails that you left out the most powerful tools you have in your communication which is your tone of voice and your body language.

The best way to engage the latter two is to use also visualization and anchoring.

If you employ visualization alongside positive affirmations, then you have got a really powerful combination at your disposal.

Furthermore, it is pertinent to pay attention to negative thoughts and beliefs when delivering your positive affirmations together with your visualization.

I strongly believe that this book "POSITIVE AFFIRMATION" is all you need to live a more positive and enjoyable life.

Thanks for your time.

List of Books written by Dr. Louise Lily Wain

Chakra Healing For Beginners: A Complete Guide to Awakening, Clearing, Unblocking and Balancing your Chakras and Your Life Through Guided meditations, Crystals, the Power of Affirmations and Yoga

Reiki Healing for Beginners: A step-by-step guide to Heal your Life, Improve your Health, and increase your Energy. Reiki Guided Meditations, Distance Healing, Working with Crystals and on Pets

Empath Healing: A survival guide to Stop Absorbing Negative Energies and Healing from Emotional Manipulation and Narcissistic abuse. Become an empowered empath by strengthening your own empathy

Master Your Emotions: Rewire Your Mind, Manage Your Feelings, Overcome Negativity, Reduce Anxiety, Stress, Anger, Worry, Develop Self-Control, and Live a Happier Life

Emotional Intelligence for Leadership: Improve Your Skills to Succeed in Business, Manage People, and Become a Great Leader — Boost Your EQ and Improve Social Skills, Self-Awareness and Charisma.

How to Analyze People: The art of reading people, discover various personality types and patterns, understand human behavior, learn types of body language and how to refrain from manipulating people.

Influence Human Behavior: Mind Control Techniques and Principles of Persuasion to be more likable, more persuasive, more confident, win friends, influence people and avoid manipulation

CPSIA information can be obtained
at www.ICGtesting.com
Printed in the USA
BVHW040752180321
602758BV00028B/110